Energetics

Energetics

Clarence M. Agress, M.D.

Grosset & Dunlap
A *Filmways Company*
Publishers   New York

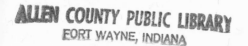

Dedication

To my dear wife, Patricia, who inspired and encouraged me to write this book, and to my ninety-four year old mother who discovered jogging and diet for herself more than fifty years ago.

Contents

Preface

Energetics, the science of energy, is derived from the Greek word for "active." It means to invigorate, to vitalize, to transform work into power. In 500 B.C., the seer Suttapitaka said, ". . .better to live one day of steadfast energy than a hundred years idle, without it. . ." Hermann von Helmholtz, the German scientist and author of *The Principle of Conservation of Force*, stated that "the quantity of force in Nature is just as eternal and unalterable as the quantity of matter." Sir Thomas Powel Buxton, the English social reformer (1786–1845), said, "The longer I live, the more deeply I am convinced that that which makes the difference between one man and another—between the weak and the powerful, the great and the insignificant—is Energy."

There is a life force in every one of us which can provide health, good spirits, and the vigor to pursue our goals. In my many years of medical practice, the most frequent complaint I hear from patients is, "I'm always so tired." Most of the time, this state is not due to a lack of vitamins, sluggish thyroid, low blood sugar, improper diet, excessive stress, or disease but rather to inadequate or improper habits of exercise. The feelings of well-being, tranquillity, enthusiasm, and joy for living don't come from any single source. However, one thing is basic: You must use your muscles. Energetics will teach you, at any age, whether you're healthy or a heart victim, to harness this inner vital force through exercise. Best of all, exercise will be a source of fun, companionship, and confidence.

A word of caution. Do not reach for a racket, do not put on jogging shoes, do not go streaking through the morning mist or engage in any other intense activity without having had a complete physical examination and exercise test. Without them, you may be courting disaster.

Acknowledgments

I wish first to express my appreciation to Mrs. Nancy Brault, librarian at St. John's Hospital in Santa Monica, California, for her untiring help in searching out the hundreds of references in the vast literature on exercise. I want to thank George Glass for his pithy comments in the preparation of the manuscript. Most of all I want to acknowledge my indebtedness to those indefatigable scientists whose researches in physiology and medicine have extended and enriched the lives of us all.

It is impossible to become nearer to God by any other way than by way of knowledge—therefore I have wished to write this book for the humble to read. Because since no book is written without reproach. . .so neither will this one be. But all the same, I implore those who see it not gnaw it with an envious tooth, but to read it through humbly, for nothing is set down here but what has been proved by personal experience either of myself or others. . .

John of Gaddesden, 1350

Introduction

The conviction that exercise is healthful and prolongs life can be traced back to many old civilizations. Maimonides, who lived in the twelfth century, advocated exercise to the point of breathlessness. Our evolutionary survival, which depended on violent effort, established patterns by natural selection for untold generations. Such patterns cannot be neglected by the machine-age, low-energy output habits of modern society without dire consequences.

In recent years, increasing recognition has been given in both medical and lay publications to the importance of exercise in the preservation of health. Witness the popularity of jogging and the amazing growth of tennis and similar sports, not only by the young but by middle-aged and older persons. Despite these trends, only a small percentage of our population participates in such activities, and, unfortunately, those who need it most are those who exercise least. Millions of our citizens are obese, diabetic, hypertensive, smokers, heart patients, or are prematurely senile. Yet most of these people could preserve their health if they followed a few simple precautionary measures. But how do you get them to do these things? Many will walk and some will run, but most are discouraged by boredom, the hazards of traffic, or loneliness.

What is not generally recognized, even by many physicians, is that the exercise programs traditionally prescribed are too exacting and fatiguing for the average man or woman—they don't produce the sense of exhilaration to make the exercise self-perpetuating. *Energetics* is just a word, but it represents a method with which you can get this feeling of vigor joyfully and sensibly, so that it will become a way of life. This book will show you how *you* can do it yourself, using scientific principles that have been firmly established by the greatest students of exercise physiology.

Energetics uses the principle of *Dash Training*, whereby energy reserves are stimulated but strain and undue fatigue are avoided. Dash Training, also called Interval Training, is a form of interrupted, rather than continuous, exercise; that is, periods of vigorous activity are alternated with periods of lesser activity. If you run a mile, that's continuous exercise, but if you run three minutes then walk three minutes for the same distance, you will be less fatigued, achieve as good or better training effect, and still reach the level of exercise required to help protect you against blood vessel diseases.

Dash Training allows most people to safely engage in sports. And because of the exhilaration and social interaction generated, many are encouraged to exercise often enough and long enough for it to become a pleasurable as well as a heart-protecting and health-promoting way of life.

I have been tremendously impressed with the concept of Dash Training and its unique suitability for achieving physical fitness for young and old—even for the heart patient. Perhaps the greatest credit should go to Drs. Per-Olof Astrand and Kaare Rodahl from Sweden, two eminent exercise physiologists whose work tables are still the Bible for all exercise books and experts in the field of physical education.

Energetics treats tennis as the prototype of this technique because it is the most popular sport in the world today and because it encompasses all the requirements of Dash Training. Special studies were made to see if older people and patients with heart disease could play tennis with reasonable safety. It was determined that this activity really was an effective training tool. These investigations, carried out on the tennis court with special devices to record heartbeat, did indeed demonstrate that tennis is an ideal Dash Training exercise. If the participant is properly tested and conditioned, he can play it most of his life and accomplish two goals at the same time: better health for the arteries and more fun for the soul.

There are many sports and exercise regimens that accomplish the same results as the racket sports. What you learn here will apply to all of them. You won't need any tables; your pulse will be your guide (see "How to Find and Count Your Own Pulse," page 31). Thus you can exercise at a level which is effective with maximum safety. You *can* become an athlete—often even after having a heart attack.

Is Exercise Healthful or Dangerous?

Pseudoscientific books and articles have held contradictory opinions as to the wisdom of exercise. Confusion abounds over what constitutes proper exercise for the normal person and for the patient with heart disease. There is great uncertainty about what training is needed for physical fitness and what can be done through exercise to retard the advance of heart disease. How much exercise does it take to be fit and how much is required to retard disease of the arteries?

Playboy magazine features an article called "Jogging Can Kill You," while *Runners World* stoutly asserts that one must run like a deer in pursuit of health and happiness. One book assures you that very little exercise is enough, while another wants you to act like the Tarahumara Indians of Mexico, whose traditions include running over one hundred miles without stopping, and who can actually catch deer and other game by running them down.

Other articles in various publications, mostly devoid of supportive study or corroborating facts, trumpet the virtues of swimming, skating, rope jumping, and calisthenics. Not that these are bad; it is just that, too often, the claims are not based upon proper research or scientific evidence. Add to this a plague of screwball fads (there are as many fads as there are faddists) from exotic herbs to mountainous ingestions of vitamins A to Z.

There is also a great amount of confusion about the hazards of exercise, particularly for those in middle or later life and for the heart patient. The need to clarify what the risks are and how they may be minimized has been either ignored or glossed over. Is there a great hazard in sudden effort or in sex? You will find the answers in this book.

What Should You Believe?

The role of diet, with and without exercise, is the most confused and controversial subject of all. Cholesterol is now a household word. The purveyors of unsaturated fats and egg substitutes have taken advantage of the terror struck in many hearts by this word. It is time that the public understand that these are theories only, still challenged after sixty-four years of extensive human and animal experiments and mass-population studies. There is no real evidence that foods like eggs cause heart attacks.

What about vitamins? The Harvard University Department of Nutrition does not recommend daily supplements believed in so passionately by unreasoning food faddists like my wife's "tennis ladies": vitamin B, wheat germ oil, vitamin E, gelatin, and phosphates. And there is no need to take salt when exercising unless one is exposed to extremely hot and dry conditions and is engaging in prolonged arduous work. It *is* important to restrict alcohol and tobacco. It is time to ask, "What's the evidence? How do *I* know that *you* know what you are talking about? I can read two opposite views in the same newspaper. The ads say, 'Eat this; Don't eat that.' Who is right?" In every day's mail there is a clipping from some patient about a new diet, a new all-curative pill, a new health program, a new spa or ranch where all your lifelong diseases are reversed in a month or less by a new diet and exercise kick.

I present in this book scientific evidence as well as my own observation and research of twenty-five years. The object is to clear away the confusion and to arrive at a consensus about exercise that is the latest proven word. The expertise of those listed in the Bibliography represents a treasury of findings about your fitness and your heart. Of course, new discoveries and research may challenge some of these conclusions, but I doubt that many will fall apart.

Just a Few Statistics

A 1976 statistical survey showed that over 1,200,000 Americans suffer heart attacks each year, many under the age of sixty-five, and 660,000 die, half without any previous indication of heart disease. Last year $118.5 billion were spent for health in the United States, along with $4 billion in disability allowances for heart attack.

Our greatest health problem is the physical fitness of our citizens. Nearly 29 million Americans have some form of heart or blood vessel disease. Many of our public health experts feel that a well-practiced physical fitness program could increase life expectancy by at least ten years. Yet the President's Council on Physical Fitness and Sports reports that 45 percent of American adults do not exercise at all.

Life expectancy for babies born in the United States in 1975 was 68.5 years for boys and 76.4 years for girls, the highest ever recorded by the National Center for Health Statistics. One hundred years ago, it was 38.3 for males and 40.5 for females. Part of the change is due to the decline in infant mortality. Although part is also due to decreased numbers of heart attacks, strokes, and auto accidents, heart disease is still the leading killer, causing more than one-third of the 1,910,000 deaths recorded in 1975.

More men than women die of cardiovascular disease each year: 413.7 men per 100,000 as compared to 228.1 women. In the United States alone, 450,000 persons die each year of sudden death from heart attack, accounting for some 25 percent of all deaths, and over 100,000 occur in people between the ages of twenty and sixty-four. It has been estimated by an impressive panel of outstanding cardiologists, in a seminar held by the International Medical Corporation, that 80 percent of the people who die from heart attacks, with no previous record of such problems, could have been diagnosed by an exercise electrocardiogram, and that at least 50 percent of these could have been saved. An estimated 20 percent of the population is vulnerable to this disease, and many are dying needlessly.

Effort Sports Are Tranquillizing

Sports medicine has been emphasized much more in European publications than in American writings, and this is surprising in a society where the leisure class is large and the average person has more money to spend on pleasures. The tranquillizing effects of sports are well known, and the physical improvement is a publicized health measure. Physicians should lend the weight of their influence to physical educators in this endeavor. The Harvard Fatigue Laboratory was established in 1947, and though it terminated ten years later, it began a new chapter in the study of exercise in this country. While studies at the Carnegie Institute began as early as 1913, in the next three decades most of the publications on the subject came out of Germany and Scandinavia.

Sports medicine has today assumed great prominence. National symposiums are held to exchange ideas among specialists in the field. The great contribution to mental health as well as to physical well-being from sports is generally accepted. Moreover, the use of sports training for the rehabilitation of the cardiac patient is also gaining greater acceptance.

Energetics

PART I
Energetics

*. . .There is a friction (bodily change) which comes after
exercise and is called rest-inducing friction. The object
of this is the resolution of superfluities retained in the
muscles. . .that they may be evaporated, and that
fatigue may not occur. . .*

Avicenna, Arabian philosopher and physician, c. 1020 AD

Chapter 1.
Dash Training

The concept of Dash or Interval Training, that is, intermittent rather
than continuous activity, was introduced by a Swedish exercise
physiologist, Per-Olof Astrand, in 1960. His research showed that optimal
amounts of blood are pumped by the heart during short bursts of activity
(work periods) alternated with rest periods of equal or shorter duration.

The alternation of short work periods of thirty seconds with equal rest
periods, or similar short hard-and-easy stresses like run-walk sequences,
will challenge the cardiovascular system and lungs; but the alternation will
not produce the strains caused by uninterrupted work over a similar length
of time. When the work periods have become longer—two to three
minutes—the subject's performance level reaches near maximum and is
performed only with great strain.

Astrand was invited as the guest of honor of a national symposium on
exercise in 1973. In his closing remarks he stated:

> My program of exercise must be the perfect program! I take my car
> to a golf course, but I do not play golf. Because it is wonderful
> terrain, I warm up, jog and walk for five minutes uphill (only
> twenty-five steps but at maximum speed) because I think it good
> training for trunk muscles and leg muscles. I walk down and
> repeat about five, six, seven times. . . .Then there is the condition-
> ing of the cardiovascular system with three minutes of running.
> Probably I could run this distance within two or two and a half
> minutes, but I think it is as effective to do it in three minutes. Rest-
> ing, jogging, and walking, and again running, are then repeated,

and after about a half-hour I am back to my car and go home. I try to devote three thirty-minute sessions per week to such training.

Dash Training causes less fatigue. This is an important practical concept because it means one can perform heavy work without overtaxing the circulation and with a *minimum of fatigue*. Training of large muscles like those in the arms and legs is accomplished just as in steady exercise, without overloading the lungs or the heart. Short work periods of thirty seconds, alternated with equal or shorter rest periods, produce excellent training results—whether for an athlete's regimen or for the rehabilitation of the convalescent patient. And this activity permits older patients to continue physically heavy jobs despite their diminishing capacity to burn oxygen. Longer periods of heavy work will inevitably produce fatigue, which comes from the creation of an "oxygen debt"—a shortage that must be paid back. With interrupted exercise, this oxygen lack is avoided because there is more time to breathe.

Recovery is faster in Dash Training. Heart rate is a reliable measure of the amount of oxygen consumed and work performed. Continuous exercise, compared to an equal amount of intermittent exercise, requires *twice* as many heartbeats during the recovery period, indicating the greater strain involved. Maximum heart rates are also less, with the same amount of work, for discontinuous exercise. The longer the work duration, even with equal-length pauses, the higher the heart rate.

Comparison of Interrupted and Continuous Exercise

Other investigations have shown that Dash Training such as running at full speed uphill for thirty to sixty seconds, repeated five to ten times and allowing low-level exercise between dashes, will improve performance. (Obviously, this kind of activity is for research only and not recommended for you sports people. We don't want to lose you this early in the game.) In ten independent studies, normal subjects as well as patients with coronary heart disease were made to perform interrupted and continuous exercises. None exercised less than thirty minutes per day for five days a week. All exhibited greatly improved performance. In many other analyses carried out in the Scandinavian countries, where the greatest interest in exercise training seems to exist, the same results as from exercise training by more fatiguing methods were reported: decreased heart rate and blood pressure, increased pumping of blood, and the like.

Edward L. Fox and associates at the Exercise Physiology and Aviation Medicine Research Laboratories at Ohio State University have analyzed untrained students by measuring heart rates, oxygen uptake by muscle and heart pumping under different methods of training: high-intensity, short-distance sprints, and low-intensity, long-distance runs. On thirty minutes of such training five days per week, the working capacity of young people increased 10 to 20 percent, and *Interval Training* (high-intensity) *was more effective in improving performance* as measured by the ability to take up oxygen, which we call aerobic power. Fitness, once achieved, can be maintained by such exercise every third day. Older groups fare similarly but at lesser degrees of performance.

Intensity of exercise, not duration, determines aerobic (or oxygen-using) power. If you train by any of three methods—short-distance fast sprints, repeated; long-distance slow runs, repeated; or both alternating equally—your ability to burn oxygen will improve. But the most effective method is repeated, short-distance, fast sprints, in which your muscles, making up 40 percent of your body weight, develop a better capacity to use oxygen and gain greater strength. In an investigation of military conscripts in Sweden, Dr. H. G. Knuttgen and associates at the Department of Physiology at Karolinska Hospital, Stockholm, and the University Hospital, Uppsala, found that very efficient training was achieved by three fifteen-minute sessions per week of three-minute exercise periods alternating with three-minute rest periods. It was concluded that physical fitness could be markedly and rapidly improved by Interval Training, and that remarkable improvement in aerobic power could be obtained in a very short time—even one month.

Not all investigators are agreed on the best exercise-rest intervals, but there is no doubt about the excellent training achieved with high-intensity exercise alternated with rest or moderate exercise: Dash Training. Another very important difference between continuous exercise like jogging and interval exercise like run-walk sequences is that in the former, a fatigue-causing oxygen debt may be built up. Much larger quantities of high-intensity work can be performed intermittently than continuously. This fact is felt to be the main reason for the success of Dash Training.

Dash Training for Heart Disease

In many of the subjects who had coronary disease, there were many indications of improved heart function due to Dash Training. The most important improvement was the attainment of a slow heart rate, which gives the heart more time to receive blood between beats. Four investigations included thirty men with coronary disease, who engaged in gradually increasing intensity of exercise. Several patients with heart pains were entirely relieved, and all were able to perform much more work. The intermittent loads included alternate running and walking and were comparable to the stresses often encountered in sports like tennis, particularly after conditioning permitted much heavier work loads. In short, Dash Training accomplished at least the results achieved by continuous training. Dr. Terrence Kavanaugh, medical director of The Toronto Cardiac Rehabilitation Center, found interval training to be a practical method of gaining aerobic power, particularly in those patients who, because of extensive disease or angina (heart pain), were unable to perform continuous training. Not all investigators agree on the relative merits of the two methods of training; both have their place and both require that the intensity and duration of the work and recovery periods or the period of continuous exercise maintain the required pulse rate.

Vigorous weekend exercise protects against heart attack. An extensive study was performed in England on 16,882 British male office workers aged forty to forty-four during the years 1968 to 1973. The subjects kept detailed records of their activities on weekends. By 1973, 232 of them had had heart attacks. Each was compared with two other subjects in the study who had remained well and who were matched in terms of smoking and coronary-risk factors. The activities of the men were analyzed. The "heavy workers" performed work equivalent to 7½ calories per minute. These were efforts like swimming, digging, and vigorous calisthenics. Those who engaged in such activities had one-third the number of heart attacks compared to those doing light exercise, where no advantage was gained. "Vigorous exercise apparently protected against rapidly fatal heart attacks and other first clinical attacks of coronary disease alike, throughout middle age," concluded Dr. J. H. Morris and associates of the London School of Hygiene and Tropical Medicine in reporting on the study.

Of particular interest was the concept of interrupted intense activity as opposed to steady activity; that is, the objective was to determine whether short peaks of activity had more of a protective effect on the cardiovascular system than continuous energy expenditure. These peaks had to approach the maximal heart rate, or energy level, of which the subject was capable. Such exercises as tennis, swimming, and hill climbing qualified. Digging, felling trees, moving heavy objects, and running could also be included, as were the Canadian Air Force calisthenics. Thirty minutes of this type of exercise were minimal for protective value. In this group, the resting pulses were lower. Men in late middle life were definitely benefited. Even those who had been sedentary were protected against cardiovascular accidents by this training.

If heart disease is to be protected against by doing exercise performed during leisure time, high (peak) heart rates must be achieved. "High intensity" is the amount of exercise producing peaks of energy output (7½ calories per minute), like tennis, digging, running, cycling eleven miles per hour, and brisk walking at five miles per hour. Dancing, golfing while carrying clubs on a hilly course, and carpentry for at least thirty minutes daily are also beneficial. No value is assessed to lesser activities.

This Study Will Impress You

In 1975, Dr. Ralph S. Paffenbarger, Jr., and Wayne E. Hale of The California State Department of Health and The University of California School of Public Health studied the mortality rates of 6,351 San Francisco longshoremen in terms of their work activity over a period of twenty-two years. Their ages ranged from thirty-five to seventy-four years. The workers were found to be remarkably sedentary off the job, but at work they were classified according to their cargo loading as having heavy, moderate, and light energy output. The heavy workers had repeated periods of peak effort rather than a steady pace (55 percent of their time was spent in labor and 45 percent in rest). The mortality rate of the high-activity group was *26.9* per ten thousand work-years, whereas those for the lower energy categories were 46 and 49. Strikingly, the *sudden death rate* for the high-activity group was less than one-third that of the low-activity group—5.6 per 10,000 work-years for heavy workers, 17.8 for the others.

It would seem, therefore, that it takes heavy work to reduce the death rate. The importance of the study is that it shows that maintaining moderate work loads offers little, if any, protection against heart attack or sudden death. There is a critical level of energy output; that is, it is necessary to reach a certain peak level to influence longevity. The men who did heavy work were repeatedly performing high-energy tasks. Many investigators have stated that there is more benefit from twenty to thirty minutes of stressful work than from a day of light work. Note also that the dock workers' labors were intermittent: Dash Training.

Heavy exercise offers protection against heart disease. The benefits of heavy exercise are reduced clotting, increased size of blood vessels, reduced blood pressure and blood fat, weight loss, increased heart action, and regulation of heart rhythm. I have seen no such statistics for the sedentary way. Many sports meet the criteria for repeated peak-energy effort over a significant time period without arduous or prolonged and tedious training. Admittedly, more data will be required to prove this, but the energy levels achieved during sports activities compare favorably with work loads which have been shown to be protective. In the British study, many of the subjects played tennis or cricket or swam.

How Much Exercise Will Diminish Coronary Disease?

Dr. Herman K. Hellerstein, director of the Work Classification Clinic in Cleveland and a great pioneer in exercise rehabilitation of the heart patient, has conducted population studies on the protective effect of exercise against heart attack: high-intensity exercise did protect against heart disease, but lighter exercise did not. As a corollary, middle-aged people in such a program can derive much benefit from it. Patients with coronary disease have been made to perform various exercises, particularly run-walk sequences, which were gradually increased in intensity. A heart rate of 140 beats per minute during run-walk sequences corresponded to 80 percent of the heart rates of which the subjects were capable. Dr. Hellerstein and John P. Naughton reported that all the beneficial effects listed for exercise in normal subjects were obtained in these individuals.

The calorie-burning effects of various activities and sports are listed in the Activity Stairway of table 4 (page 37). This listing will help you to select those activities best suited to you.

I do not believe that training programs should be gauged from standard charts. There are too many variations caused by age, presence of disease, previous conditioning, and type of exercise; also, the blood pressure response or presence of abnormalities may not be known. The intensity, duration, and rate of repetition are still being studied, but there are enough facts to plan an intelligent and effective program for each individual. At the last meeting of the American Medical Joggers Association, the amount of exercise I have discussed met their requirements for significant improvement and protection. The optimum amount of running is still being argued. Some say it takes six miles per day to be effective. If this is true, I doubt that a significant portion of our population would pursue a persistent regimen; certainly the safety factor is questionable for the masses. If you do run, and, particularly, if you are past middle age, even if you have been tested, I think it is important *not to run alone*, because should an accident occur, help could come too late. This is another reason I prefer group sports.

What Can We Conclude from All These Studies?

There are at least four conclusions from all these investigations:
1. Vigorous activity like sprinting for one-half to one minute alternating with short periods of rest, or reduced activity for two to three minutes, significantly develops aerobic power. Shorter periods will strengthen tendons and ligaments, but will not increase aerobic power.
2. The exercise must involve large muscle groups like the arms and legs; it's better if both are involved.
3. The duration of the exercise period must approach a period of thirty minutes for significant development of endurance whether the exercise is steady or intermittent; both will provoke

the body to respond by increasing the ability of the tissues to extract oxygen from the blood, and by strengthening the heart as a pump.

4. Excellent training is achieved by interval exercise (dash training) with reduced fatigue because the body's oxygen needs are replenished during the rest or moderate activity periods; that is, the "oxygen debt" of steady exercise is minimized or avoided. This principle has many applications in sports and in work programs, expecially for older people.

The maintenance of health lies in forsaking the disin-
clination to exertion. Nothing is to be found that can
substitute for exercise in any way, because in exercise
the natural heat flames up and all the superfluities are
expelled, while at rest the flame of the natural heat sub-
sides and superfluities are engendered in the body, even
though the food is of the very best quality and is mod-
erate in quantity. And exercise will expel the harm done
by most of the bad regimens that most men follow.

Hippocrates, c. 420 BC

Chapter 2.
Why Exercise?

What evidence do we have that any more exercise than occurs in daily life is beneficial? Do active individuals live longer than sit-down persons? These questions are answered in a delightful book called *Youth in Old Age.* I was collecting data on longevity when I came across this book, written by Dr. Alexander Leaf, a professor of medicine at Harvard. With the aid of the National Geographic Society, Dr. Leaf had gone to the three places in the world where people live longest: Abkhasia, in the Caucasus Mountains of Georgia, Russia; Hunza, in the Karakoram Range of Kashmir; and Vilcabamba, in the Andes Mountains of Ecuador. Centenarians abound in these areas in much higher percentages than elsewhere in the world.

Although the advanced ages of 165 to 195 claimed by the Novosti Press Agency of the Soviet Union in Daghestan are unsubstantiated, Dr. Leaf was able to document ages up to 115. However, it is not the long lives of these people alone that is impressive, but the fact that they are healthy, often sexually as well as physically and intellectually active, enjoying full and rewarding lives. Interviews revealed that the factors influencing their longevity were few psychological pressures and good social influences, nutrition, heredity, and sexual and physical activity. But one characteristic stood out: These people stayed fit by vigorous exercise throughout their lives. They were digging ditches and chopping down trees at 110. Some smoked, drank, and were overweight, but none was inactive. Herein lies the answer.

What Is Human Aging?

The body is made up of little individual building blocks called cells, which wear out and duplicate themselves. The number of times they can rebuild determines how long the body—yours—lives. This ability to rebuild cells differs for humans and animals and insects. A butterfly lives a day or two; a Galapagos tortoise, 125 years, with a possible span of 175 years. The human now lives around 75 years in the United States, with a possible life span of 115 years. Alexis Carrel, a French surgeon and biologist, kept a cell culture alive for 34 years and then voluntarily terminated it. It seemed that cell immortality had been achieved. However, since 1919 no one has been able to do this except with cancer cells. Cell biologists believe that there is a little time clock in the nucleus of each cell which determines when it will no longer double. Fifty to sixty doublings account for the usual life span of human cells.

Although deterioration is inevitable, the steady increase in life expectancy we have been witnessing is due to the conquest of disease. Dr. Leonard Hayflick (of the National Institute of Aging and the National Institute of Health, Bethesda) has calculated that if we eliminate heart disease and stroke, eighteen more years of life are added; only two if cancer is eradicated. The twenty-odd years added to life expectancy in the last half-century applies to causes of death occurring before age sixty-five; from ages sixty-five to seventy-five, the expectancy increased only two to three years.

It is unlikely that scientists will be able to prolong the capacity of the cell to duplicate itself. But, some people do live to advanced ages, and—more importantly—they are enjoying life at that age. Living longer, then, means realizing our potential, not outwitting nature. That this can be done by better habits of living there is no doubt.

The specialists in this field, the gerontologists, agree that there is no single cause of aging, but they do not agree on what the many factors are. "First we ripen, and then we rot" merely affirms the dependence on that hereditary time clock, but there are other independent factors.

Dr. Charles H. Barrows, of the Gerontology Research Center, National Institute of Aging, has shown that the life span of insects can be almost doubled merely by diluting the media in which they live—reducing the food supply. Reducing the daily intake of food, chiefly protein, markedly extends the life span of rats and mice. Both caloric and protein restrictions are involved, and human experiments are now being conducted. While all this is experimental, we have long known that overeating shortens life.

Aging is a complex process during which maximal breathing capacity declines, heart vigor diminishes, capability for work lessens, and reflexes become slower. All these changes can be deferred by regular exercise, which preserves endurance, strength, and skill. Feats of endurance by older people are legion. In *Physical Activity and Aging*, E. Jokl recounts the case of a sixty-seven-year-old university professor who won the Honolulu Marathon in 1974, requiring only four hours to run twenty-six miles. He had been sedentary until his sixty-fourth year!

The only way to live a long time is to become old, but you don't have to be decrepit. I play tennis with several men in their seventies, and the quickness of their reflexes is incredible.* C. P. is a prominent dentist who has played tennis all his life and, at seventy-two, now competes with men ten to fifteen years younger than himself. I have repeatedly seen him exchange balls at the net at breakneck speed, and usually it is he who puts the ball away.

I remember an oldster, aged seventy-eight, whom I was encouraging to lead an active life. He came in one day after his golf game very discouraged about his score. I said to him, "Milton, what are you trying to do—shoot your age?" He replied, quick as a flash, "I'd be glad to shoot my blood pressure!"

Does Exercise Prolong Life?

A study of Copenhagen men aged forty to forty-nine showed lower risks for the fit, even when they were overweight and had high blood pressure, diabetes, or lung disease. The life spans of 396 Finnish champion endurance skiers born between 1845 and 1910 were followed up to 1967 by Dr. Martti J. Karvonen of Helsinki. They outlived the average male population of their generation by five to seven years. There were no differences in the cholesterol levels of these groups, but the athletes had lower blood pressures.

In the previously noted San Francisco longshoremen study, the rate of fatal coronary heart disease, and particularly sudden death, in over twenty-seven thousand man-years of heavy longshoreman work was only half as high as in men performing light work. There were no differences in the groups in relation to blood pressure, cigarette smoking, body weight, or sugar intolerance.

Dr. Edward A. Mortimer and his associates have reported an interesting observation on the coronary mortality rate of people residing at high altitudes in the Rocky Mountains. As the altitude increased, the mortality rate

---

*The time it takes to respond to a stimulus when the element of choice is involved is known as *reaction time*. For instance, a subject is instructed to raise his right hand if he sees a green light; his left hand if he sees a red light. This can be used to test the degree of aging or to measure senility. When you say, "He has good reflexes for his age," you mean he is delaying aging. Only habitual usage can do that. That's why it is not safe for some old people to drive a car; their responses are too slow to avoid an accident when a choice is involved.

declined in males but not in females. The investigators examined race, migration of ill persons, urban versus rural living, ethnic factors, cigarette smoking, and so on, and concluded that the most probable explanation was that, since adaptation to reduced amounts of oxygen at high altitudes is never complete, just the activities of daily living constituted increased exercise.

Despite the many studies of sedentary versus active types in populations of various parts of the world showing the beneficial and protective effects of exercise, there are some who say that the differences are due to other factors. In a convincing experiment, Dr. Daniel Brunner, of the Government Hospital at Jaffa, made a study of the kibbutz environment of Israel, where it was possible to separate occupation and physical effort at work from economic and life habits because all those studied lived together under the same conditions. Moreover, food was prepared for the whole community from one kitchen. There were no differences in leisure-time activities, cholesterol, or triglycerides in the active as compared to the inactive groups. Yet, in the 5,288 men and 5,229 women ranging in age from forty to sixty-four, coronary disease was 2 to 3.5 times higher in the sedentary workers.

Sitters and Walkers

Is there good evidence that people who live active physical lives do better than those who loaf? In 1958, J. N. Morris conducted his now-classic studies of London postal workers and bus drivers. Deaths of postal workers who carried mail bags were only one-third compared to those who stayed at their desks; and the sit-down drivers suffered more deaths than the fare collectors who walked up and down the double-decker buses. Morris's studies also included a national survey of Britain, which showed that physical activity did indeed protect against heart disease.

Nature's secrets are hard to come by, and simple experiments are often misleading. But Drs. S. M. Fox and W. L. Haskel reported on nine studies from 1957 to 1969 which, with one exception, showed less heart disease in those who habitually exercised. The prestigious 1948 Framingham, Massachusetts, studies (discussed in Chapter 7) of a controlled population also showed definitely lower cardiovascular disease in active subjects.

The President's Council on Physical Fitness and Sports was established in 1956 under Eisenhower. Dr. C. Carson Conrad, executive director, has long advocated the need to promote physical fitness in order to advance national health. He has pointed out that one of the chief obstacles to this is public opinion. The Summer Youth Sports Program has been made available to school-age children during the summer months, and now attention is also being directed to the elderly, who are urged to follow some program attuned to their capabilities. The motto is, "Put life in your years." Studies show that people from fifty-five to seventy-one years of age who did regular physical activity, despite a slight decline of exercise tolerance, could perform well at high work loads.

J. S. is now seventy. Every day he runs at least two miles at the UCLA track and then goes up and down the steps for ten to fifteen minutes. He plays vigorous tennis, has a resting heart rate of fifty-six, and appears ten years younger than he really is. He carries on an exacting business, is active in several important philanthropies, and has a keen, active mind.

Dr. H. K. Hellerstein, a noted authority on exercise and heart disease and a leader in the National Exercise and Heart Disease program, has followed over fifteen hundred people with and without coronary artery disease for at least seventeen years. He has found 40 percent less heart disease in those who exercised.

Can previously sedentary middle-aged and older people become conditioned? E. F. is now eighty-two years old. I first saw him twenty-two years ago for treatment of a heart murmur. He was worried about it, particularly because he enjoyed tennis and an unusually active sex life. I found a loud murmur, but otherwise he was sound. I helped him overcome his fears and encouraged him to continue his life without apprehension. He has been reexamined every year on the treadmill and still plays tennis five times a week (he eliminated singles only two years ago). And he always has a girl-friend about one-fourth his age.

On the other hand, I see patients of similar age with sedentary habits who are becoming forgetful, have little or no motivation, and are certainly getting no fun out of life.

We now have evidence that middle-aged and older people who have never exercised in their lives can become as fit as younger ones or as people who have habitually pursued vigorous activities. The National Institute of Occupational Health in Stockholm tested men from forty to sixty-three years of age for ten weeks. The subjects were put through both intermittent and continuous hard exercises. These included warm-ups, jogging, alternate running and fast walking for two-to-four minute periods, and continuous running for thirty minutes three times a week. In the intermittent-exercise group, the heart rates and oxygen uptake were near maximal; in the continuous-running groups, the subjects pushed themselves to a speed that demanded more energy than the oxygen they could take in. The results? The ability of the tissues to use oxygen increased 18 percent, independent of age; breathing power increased 51 percent. Resting and top heart rates slowed ten to sixteen beats per minute, again without regard to age; and so on, for more technical measurements. The improvement in these older men was entirely similar to that found in younger men. An important observation, also, was that the heart could perform more work with each stroke after training. This is one of the major benefits of training after heart attack, and may be one of the most important factors contributing to less coronary disease in active people.

Many recent studies of middle-aged men indicate that thirty minutes of vigorous activity three times a week produces conditioning similar to that found in younger men. In other words, it is well established that fitness can be achieved at any age in healthy subjects, and for the majority of patients with heart disease.

What About Animal Studies?

Dr. Hans Selye, professor and director of the Institute of Experimental Medicines & Surgery, Montreal, and one of the greatest authorities on stress, found that a sustained program of running protected rats against heart damage caused by stress. If rats are exercised on an inclined treadmill for twenty minutes, five days per week, at ten miles per hour, survival increases at all ages. Evidence for increase in blood supply through exercise, either by enlargement of existing channels or growth of new ones, is also a controversial subject. But consider some of this evidence:

Is the common form of artery blockage—arteriosclerosis—reversible? In several animal exercise experiments reported by Dr. R. W. Eckstein (of the Department of Medicine of Montefiore Hospital and Medical Center, New York) it was demonstrated that new channels have been formed around obstructed coronary vessels. Controlled studies on rats by Dr. J. Scheuer have established that the response of the heart to diminished oxygen supply can be greatly improved by exercise.

Over seven years ago, Dr. Mark L. Armstrong (of the Department of Internal Medicine and Pathology, University of Iowa, and Department of Medicine for Veterans Administration Hospital, Iowa City) and his associates demonstrated that manipulating the diet of the rhesus monkey over forty months caused almost complete disappearance of obstructions in diseased arteries, and that the channels through them became much less narrowed.

In March 1977, at the 26th Annual Scientific Session of the American College of Cardiology, Drs. H. L. Wyatt and J. H. Mitchell (respectively professor of medicine and physiology and director of cardiopulmonary research, Southwestern Medical School, Dallas) presented a paper on the effect of exercise on arteries in the hearts of dogs. The dogs were alternately run on treadmills or confined to cages after training. The size of the arteries was examined both by X-rays (angiograms) and by removal of a small portion of the heart muscle (biopsy). Thus both the diameter (caliber) and the cross-sectional area could be measured under the microscope. The results: Conditioning did increase the size of the arteries, which became smaller when deconditioning was induced. The authors of the paper concluded that conditioning did indeed improve the blood supply, but that regular exercise was necessary to maintain the improvement.

Relationship of Animal Studies to Humans

Clarence De Mar was a famous marathon runner who continued to compete until he was 69 and finally died of cancer. At autopsy, his heart arteries were twice the size of the average person's.

The development of new vessels (collaterals) in humans through exercise is still controversial, but all agree that the heart becomes more efficient as a pump and provides a better blood supply during increased work and becomes less susceptible to the complications of arterial disease. Drs. Robert Wissler, professor, Department of Pathology and director, SCOR-Atherosclerosis, and Dragoslava Vesselinovitch, associate professor, Department of Pathology, University of Chicago, have examined evidence that atherosclerosis is largely preventable and reversible, both in the animal and the human. Their experimental studies in the rhesus monkey showed that arterial disease like that of the human could be produced or reversed by manipulations of the fat content of the diet. Dr. Henry Buchwald of the University of Minnesota School of Medicine has shown by heart artery X-rays over a period of three years that regression of heart artery blockage occurs after removal of some of the small bowel. This procedure is used in the hopelessly obese, because they lose weight through their inability to absorb fat when this part of the intestine is removed (ileal bypass).

A good example of how the blood supply in diseased arteries can be increased by exercise is the effect of increased walking on patients with leg pain caused by narrowing arteries in their legs. These people have severe pain, usually in the calves. This pain, which is like the pain in the chest produced by coronary artery disease, occurs after walking a certain distance and may become so severe that the patient has to stop. Progressive walking has been shown to alter the chemistry of leg muscle so that it contracts more vigorously, increases in size, and can use more oxygen. Through progressive walking, patients can greatly increase the distance they are able to walk without pain, and this regimen is more effective than any known drug treatment.

P. L. is a builder. He has had a severe lack of thyroid for years, as well as coronary artery disease. He recently remarried, began to eat heavily and gained fifteen pounds, and neglected what had been a lifelong exercise program. In six months, he developed a severe episode of shortness of breath due to accumulation of fluid in his lungs. Then he began to take care of himself. He lost weight, reduced the salt in his diet, and resumed his walking program. But now he began to have severe pain in his calves, due to advancing obstruction of his calf arteries. He tried many medicines, including large doses of vitamin E, without benefit. Then he began to walk, painfully at first, and only for short distances. But he persisted. In three months, he could walk for over thirty minutes without pain and also resumed playing golf (without a cart). He now states that he never felt better in his life.

Drs. R. Barndt and David Blankenhorn of the University of Southern California have demonstrated direct visual evidence of the disappearance of disease in an artery by the technique of digital imaging, which allows X-rays of arteries to be read with ease. This method was originally developed by the Jet Propulsion Lab in Pasadena for procuring spacecraft pictures. In some patients on a program to stop smoking who exercised to achieve pulse rates of 130 to 150, deposits of calcium and cholesterol in leg arteries become measurably smaller. However, nearly two years of this program were necessary to demonstrate these improvements. The same improvements were demonstrated on heart arteries and there are other heart-artery X-ray studies showing that humans can establish new sources of blood supply, even when they have advanced disease. In these studies, the data indicated that physical activity leads to increased caliber of the coronary vessels, making the disease process less consequential.

How About People Who Already Have Heart Disease?

William Heberden, in 1772, wrote about coronary artery disease and the beneficial effects of exercise, as did Calib H. Parry in 1779. But two hundred years went by during which these observations were not only ignored but were held in disrepute. In 1955, Victor Gottheiner (of the Center for Sports Medicine, Wingate Institute of Physical Training, Tel-Aviv) started an active reconditioning program through sports training for heart attack victims in Israel. Now many investigations show that men with this disease who undertake exercise programs have less recurrence of heart attack and live longer than their nonexercising counterparts.

Three independent comparisons of sedentary with exercising persons showed a reduction of mortality in the latter. In one of them, Dr. Benjamin L. Rosen, associate director of the Cardiac Rehabilitation Program in San Pedro, California, has given examples of patients who under endurance training lose their angina and are able to achieve remarkable feats of physical strength. One patient, a male aged fifty-five, had incapacitating angina and an arteriogram that showed three-vessel disease with 90 percent blockage of all three arteries. He was advised to have heart surgery, but refused. Instead he began to train intensively, soon running several miles per day. In eight months, he competed successfully in the Hawaiian Marathon! He has not yet had another angiogram, but his treadmill test shows marked improvement. There is a remarkable case of disappearance of high blood pressure and reopening of the narrowed kidney arteries by drug treatment of blood fats. Dr. Vasta and associates took artery X-rays several years apart that showed marked reopening of the arteries after treatment.

If two people had proven coronary disease, the inactive one would have only one-quarter the chance of surviving as the one who performed the necessary amount of exercise. Maybe this kind of evidence is all you will ever have, because a completely scientific study would require very large numbers of subjects being followed for very many years, with strictly supervised control groups; that is, one group would exercise and another would not. Such strict control becomes difficult when an experiment's subjects are human. I think there is enough evidence now to tell you to go out and have fun while you improve your health.

Put Your Money on Exercise

The effects of exercise in both animals and humans are still being studied. Medicine has done about-faces on many of its opinions. For example, we used to believe that roughage was bad for the bowel, and now, because of Dr. D. P. Burkitt's work, from Medical Research Council of External Scientific Staff in London, we are all recommending fiber foods like bran for diseases of the colon so enthusiastically that supermarkets are running out of bran supplies. Dr. Andrew F. Ippoliti has shown us that milk stimulates acid formation in the stomach, and all these years we have been prescribing it for the treatment of ulcers.

Medicine was certainly very slow to recognize the very great risk of cigarette smoking. Even when the effects became known, it took ten more years before doctors got the message over to the public, because they were not thoroughly convinced themselves. We didn't recognize what a heart attack was until 1912, and it was another decade before it became general knowledge. Many of you were in high school or college before you knew that a blocked heart artery could kill you. Is it any wonder that those who do not critically examine the facts will argue about the benefits of exercise?

Admittedly, among medical authorities, prolongation of life by exercise is still a controversial subject. Advocates on either side will argue for years to come. Blaise Pascal, the great mathematician and philosopher of the seventeenth century, decided that it was better to believe in God and the hereafter and enjoy the prospect during one's existence than to deny what could not be proved and live in doubt. And even if life is not prolonged, no one will deny that keeping fit adds greatly to the zest and enjoyment of our years.

In reviewing what has happened to my heart patients over the past twenty-five years, there is no doubt in their minds or mine of the marvelous benefits of the vigorous life. They feel better. Arteriographers, in performing angiograms on older people, have always been amazed at the extent of the extra (collateral) channels they have developed. Even when heart surgery eventually became necessary (as may happen even in those who exercise), the large run-off vessels below the points of obstruction have greatly facilitated the success of bypass operations (in which new arteries are spliced into the heart).

Lung Disease and Exercise Training

While the emphasis here has been on diseases of the circulatory system, many exercises and sports are invaluable for the treatment of respiratory diseases. Skiing, bicycling, swimming, rowing—all are great activities that help us escape the smog and dust of the cities. Both bronchitis and emphysema improve with these exercises. Breathing exercises should be performed by those more severely affected, and can be done while hiking or cycling. Volleyball can often be played with enjoyment by the emphysema patient. While the training value is low, golf, croquet, archery, billiards, skeetshooting and the like provide pleasant recreational benefits. Patients with asthma are particularly rewarded by sports, especially when the Dash Training principle of activity and rest at appropriate intervals is observed. Probably the best lung-training exercise is swimming, because the water pressure on the chest forces increased expiration.

There are some asthmatics whose attacks are brought on by exercise, and in some young people, exercise may be the only time wheezing occurs. Loss of heat and moisture through rapid breathing is believed to be the cause, and experiments show that such episodes can be prevented by breathing warm, moist air. I have found that here also swimming is the best exercise for such asthmatics.

Aging is often manifested by the restrictive effect on the lungs caused by the formation of microscopic scarring. The ability to expand the chest and take in oxygen slowly is reduced until the "vital capacity" lessens to the point where even small exertions cause shortness of breath. I know of no way to combat this except through breathing or other exercises.

Benefits of Exercise

The great astronomer, Johannes Kepler, once said, "Something can be proved only when it can be measured." The following benefits, compiled by physiologists and cardiologists, have been measured and are a direct result of vigorous exercise, even in as short a period as twelve weeks of training.

TABLE 1
Benefits of Exercise

Increased	*Decreased*
Ability of heart to pump (4-fold)	Resting heart rate
Ability of heart to pump more per stroke	Exercise heart rate
Ability of blood to carry oxygen (12-fold)	Blood pressure
Blood flow to muscles (18-fold)	Heart size (for same amount of work)
Ease of blood flow (by thinning)	Blood clots (especially in legs)
Caliber and number of heart arteries	Irregular heart rhythms
Resting time between heartbeats (more time for flow through heart)	Requirement for oxygen
Depth and calm of breathing	Recovery time from exertion
Coordination	Reaction time
Lean body weight	Fat tissue (obesity)
Sexual activity	Appetite
Tolerance to stress	Anxiety, depression, and hypochondriasis
Sense of well-being	Smoking
Tranquillity	Tension
Confidence	Cholesterol (LDL)
Strength	Triglycerides
Return to normal electrocardiogram	Sugar intolerance

If man were to conduct himself as he manages the animal he rides, he would be safeguarded from many ailments. That is, you find no one who throws fodder to his animal haphazardly, but rather he measures it out to her, so that she does not stand still forever and be ruined. Yet he does not do this for himself, or pay attention to the exercise of his own body, which is the cornerstone of the conservation of health and the repulsion of most ailments.

Maimonides, 1198

Chapter 3.
How Much Exercise?

An untold number of people really have nothing wrong with them but are deteriorating from overweight and lack of exercise. Perhaps you are a middle-aged or older person who wants to play tennis but have never done anything even as strenuous as pushing yourself away from the table. It may be that you are actually afraid of exercise.

Many health clubs, YMCAs, and the like, with trained physical educators, do excellent jobs of training the deconditioned and raising the level of physical fitness. There are the Canadian Air Force exercises; devices advertised on television; home treadmills or bicycles; pedaling machines and so forth. Heart associations now foster rehabilitation programs for patients who are recovering from heart attacks.

One often hears statements to the effect that physical conditioning can be achieved by very small expenditures of time and effort. These time periods are claimed to be as short as twenty minutes a week or even one minute a day. Such statements usually have little or no factual basis. The public has no way of knowing what to believe and is apt to be impressed by whatever purports to offer spectacular results while being so temptingly easy. Scientific observation is difficult enough to evaluate. Cicero, long before P. T. Barnum, said that it is easy to fool those who wish to be deceived. Think of the people you know who go for tonics, megavitamins, and health foods in that eternal Ponce de Leon search for the elixir of life, which, like the bluebird of happiness, is in your own backyard—your body.

The Bibliography contains a sampling from an overwhelming body of literature on the research of the world's great laboratories. It is these authorities I quote in discussing the amount of exercise that has been found to produce a proper degree of fitness.

Here's What the Real Experts Say

Many young and middle-aged adults have been studied to determine the amount of exercise needed to achieve conditioning and to maintain it. *Physical fitness* is defined in terms of the work performed (calories burned per minute) as compared to the individual's abilities at the outset. Obviously, the less fit have greater room for improvement. Each period of exercise involves a warm-up time (calisthenics, running, and the like) necessary to raise the pulse to around 120 beats per minute. This is followed by a period of exertion approaching the individual's submaximal capacity; that is, below the point where collapse from exhaustion might occur. This preserves the safety factor.

The authorities on this subject have found that the *minimum effective exercise* (vigorous but not all-out) is *thirty minutes three times a week*. It helps to supplement this by walking at every opportunity, substituting stairs for elevators, and similar activities. Five sessions per week of sixty minutes each will lead to a 50 percent improvement in about eight weeks. In middle-aged men, one hour three days a week was required to alter death rates. Three twenty-minute sessions of intense exercise per week will maintain fitness.

I have personal communications from five noted physicians who are directors of physical training programs, and all state that the *minimal* amount of exercise that will maintain basic cardiorespiratory health and endurance is thirty minutes at least three times per week at no lower than 80 percent of an individual's working capacity. None has been able to identify any sound basis for claims of significant fitness being achieved in any less time. If you train below 50 percent of your maximal aerobic power (oxygen burned), you will not improve at all.

In young subjects, a treadmill run of thirty minutes each day for one month does not cause improvement if the heart rate is under 135 a minute. Training athletes to high levels of performance may require heart rates of 174 to 198.

Studies have shown that short periods of exercise performed only one to two days per week will produce a certain degree of conditioning. Fifteen percent improvement was obtained in an eight-week program involving only thirty minutes of exercise once a week. Similar results were obtained in middle-aged men who exercised at 80 to 90 percent of their maximal heart rates for forty-five minutes twice a week. It would seem that the person playing tennis three times a week will benefit provided the exercise is vigorous enough to elevate the heart rate to 80 percent of the maximal level. This level is a function of age as well as training (see next chapter).

Individualization Is the Best Way

It is important to remember that standardized charts and tables are generalizations, and every individual is different. Even when tests are carried out during strictly standardized conditions, there is considerable error in the prediction of aerobic power. Such things as infections, a recently eaten meal, previous engagement in work, smoking, outside temperature and humidity all affect the results of any test. Heart rate (see Appendix C) may be a better criterion of performance capacity, even if fear, excitement, or other emotional stress is present. Finally, it is *absolutely necessary* to know the *blood pressure* attained to truly evaluate any performance test.

It should be emphasized that those who exercise several times a week achieve higher levels of physical fitness than those who exercise sporadically. Of course, the amount of time spent greatly influences the end result.

Duration of exercise must take age into consideration. The length of an exercise period is highly correlated with age but is not significantly different for each sex. Appendix C (page 139) shows you how to calculate the expected duration of exercise for your age. If you cannot do at least 70 percent of this value, your exercise capacity is too low for the type of exercise you are doing.

For exercise to be valuable in terms of conditioning, then, it must be of sufficient duration; it must be intense enough to raise the heart rate to a certain level; and it must involve large muscles like those of the limbs.

Progressive walking is an excellent way to begin training. One starts at one's own pace, gradually increasing the time and distance until a fifteen-mile-an-hour speed is reached and three miles are covered—three miles in forty-five minutes. Most people are well conditioned at this point. Some of my heart patients have been doing this at least three hundred days a year for over twenty years, and most of them enjoy the walk and feel exhilarated by it (see chapter 8, "Rehabilitation of the Heart Attack Patient").

Interestingly, people naturally select three miles per hour as their walking speed because the most efficient caloric cost is achieved at this rate. More work is required to walk a given distance at slow speeds than at ordinary speeds! Most people cannot walk faster than five miles per hour, and have to run to attain higher speeds. It takes less energy to run than to walk at speeds higher than five miles per hour! Other factors also increase the work load: the grade (uphill), wearing heavy or high-heeled shoes, uneven ground, tight clothing. Arm exercise is more work than leg exercise;

you can tell that if you jump rope. Racket sports use both the arms and the legs.

A trained athlete's heart is capable of pumping about 4½ quarts of blood per minute (about twenty times the resting value), or working at a level of two horsepower. Even such athletes accumulate an "oxygen debt," measured by determining the amount of waste product, known as lactic acid, which accumulates in the muscles. Since recovery may take an hour or more, depending on the degree of conditioning, it is not surprising that one feels fatigued after hard exercise.

How Do Great Athletes Do It?

Studies have been made of top athletes to find out why such people are capable of superior performances. Dr. Peter Cavanagh of Pennsylvania State University has studied the muscle and energy systems of the famous marathon runners. He worked with men like Dr. Mike Pollock, director of the Institute for Aerobics Research, and Dr. David Costell, of the Ball State University Human Performance Laboratory. They confirm the "slow and fast twitch" of muscle fibers—the slow for long distance and the fast for short energy outputs—and the tremendous ability of the runners to increase the amount of oxygen that can be utilized at maximum exercise. This was far higher than the average fit person can attain. In addition, the athletes were much more efficient; that is, they were like a car that can get more mileage per gallon. How they do this is so far unexplained, but it's probably a combination of inheritance and training. Exercise physiologists are experimenting with high-energy foods and the like to increase the performance of Olympic-type athletes. One method is for the athlete to adapt to a high altitude, where he produces more blood due to the rarified air, then bring him to sea level; then to withdraw some of the blood and transfuse his own red blood cells just before an endurance contest. So far this is legal but its value is controversial.

Male Hormone for Athletes

Around 1960 many athletes, particularly weight lifters, began taking a male hormone called methandrostenolone (Dianabol®) in the belief that it improved their strength and performance. There is some evidence that weight and even strength may be improved; perhaps fatigue is diminished and injuries heal faster. But Dr. A. V. Knibbs and associates substituted sugar pills in the same men and produced similar results; the weight gain was shown to be largely water. However, even when there is an initial gain in strength it is replaced in six weeks by weakness. And this is often accompanied by acne, decreased sexual desire, high blood pressure, bleeding from the bowel, headache, and the like. It is still being used in large amounts by an unknown number, probably large, despite the harmful effects and the efforts of sports authorities to ban such drugs. In Britain these drugs are black market items. It is unfortunate that athletes are subjected to such pressures that they must take drugs that are potentially harmful.

What You Can Do

Warming up, like a pitcher about to go into the box, is necessary before beginning exercise. When one is walking, the warm-up is automatic. For other forms of exercise, it is necessary to allow the muscles and the cardiovascular system to adapt gradually to an increasing degree of exertion. All kinds of physiological responses take place: the blood flow redistributes to the muscles and other vital areas; the lungs take in more oxygen; the heart increases its rate and stroke power; the muscles are supplied with more energy from materials like sugar and adrenalin. About ten minutes is required for adequate warm-up, and an equal time should be spent in cooling down before you jump into a shower.

It is important to remember that weather, particularly high humidity, smog, heat or cold, and clothing preventing heat loss put more stress on the exerciser. Strenuous exercise should never be undertaken until at least one and preferably two hours after a meal. This includes cold drinks, coffee, alcohol, and smoking.

Although keeping to a well-balanced diet is important, the relative size or composition of a meal does not influence athletic performance. Three to five high-carbohydrate meals per day taken for several days before a contest is said to heighten the abilities of an endurance athlete, but it is not important to the average person. Protein intake does not influence performance.

The Sports Medical Foundation of America, sponsored by the American Medical Association, has recently published a manual called *The Medical Aspects of Sports.* Fifteen percent of the diet they recommend is derived from protein; 35 percent from fat; and 50 percent from carbohydrate. All nutrient requirements are met by food; no vitamin or mineral supplements are required. Complete diets are given in the manual which you can obtain from AMA, Order Department OP-452, 535 N. Dearborn Street, Chicago, Illinois 60610.

The Foundation recommends that meals be eaten three hours before exercise, particularly in a competitive event. A sample meal is composed of 2 ounces of roast beef, ½ cup of mashed potatoes, a dinner roll with margarine, ½ cup of carrots, 8 ounces of milk, 4 ounces of orange juice, ½ cup of canned peaches, and 2 cookies (750 calories). One and one-half cups of fruit juice every hour during games will support energy and combat dehydration. Avoid sugar and candy, which pull fluid into the gut and tend to dehydrate. Taking frequent sips of water during exertion also combats dehydration, but don't drink large quantities at one time.

The American Heart Association has explicitly warned that the greater the exertion and the older the patient, the more necessary it is to evaluate the kind of exercise contemplated. Obviously, in prescribing exercise—and it *is* a prescription which must be individually determined—a physician makes entirely different recommendations for young normal people, middle-aged or old normal people, and for patients with different types and degrees of heart disease. The doctor does this by clinical evaluation based on a careful history and a physical examination. Most patients do not appreciate the skill required in taking a good medical history. It is often worth more than the most elaborate tests.

Many people believe that strenuous exercise is dangerous and should be avoided, expecially by those of middle age or older. That they feel this way is not surprising. In the nineteenth century, many doctors wrote of "heart strain" and "athletic heart" being caused by organized games. In 1898, Sir Lauder Brunton wrote on the "vulnerability of the heart" of young boys. It was not until 1935 that F. W. Lempriere jarred the medical profession by his conclusion, from a thirty-year study of sixteen thousand school boys, that it was not possible to strain the heart of a normal young person through exercise. Since then, the sports achievements of our young men and women have been little short of miraculous.

There is no such thing as "athletic heart." Part of the confusion has arisen because an enlarged heart is usually regarded as a diseased heart; yet the heart of the highly trained athlete *is* larger than the average person's because it is a very well-developed muscle with unusual strength and a large capacity to propel an increased amount of blood with each beat. On the other hand, very sedentary people have small hearts ("loafer's heart"). When athletes with large hearts give up their hard training, their hearts decrease in size, usually to normal.

There are some who have questioned the wisdom of developing a larger heart through exercise, although this change takes place only in superathletes such as marathon runners. The argument is that, because the muscle is bigger, it might not have a sufficient blood supply. Dr. Paul White, professor emeritus of Medicine, Harvard, who did not believe this, called this the "porpoise heart," because the heart of this mammal is quite large in proportion to its body size. A recent study of this question of "athletic heart" has concluded that superior performance was achieved and that the changes were entirely beneficial.

Combustion is not the result of the liberation of phlogiston but is the result of the combination of the burning substance with oxygen...

Antoine Laurent Lavoisier, 1777

Chapter 4.
How Heart Work Is Measured

Since 1789, when Antoine Lavoisier first measured the amount of oxygen being consumed by the body, there have been various methods for measuring the amount of work performed during exercise. Basically, they are measurements of the amount of energy required, particularly the amount of energy burned, which is measured in calories. The simplest method is to count the heart rate, because it has been demonstrated by many investigators that the heartbeat reflects the amount of oxygen being burned or the amount of heart work being performed. Your degree of physical fitness can be determined by the amount of oxygen you are able to burn and is reflected by your heart rate.

The highest recorded oxygen consumption in a supermarathon runner was 82 ml/kg/min (milliliters/kilogram/minute). An average jogger burns 50 ml, a sedentary person, 25 ml, and a severely diseased heart victim, 10 ml.

The heart rate (your pulse), then, can be used as a measure of an individual's training progress. The rate gradually decreases at a given load as the circulatory capacity is improved, and the heart rate of a person, compared to the same person's previously determined rate, is a more valuable index than reference to a table of averages. As the body gradually adapts to training, greater work loads are necessary to achieve higher levels of fitness. The older the individual, the less trainable he or she is, but some effect can be achieved even in very old age.

You will hear a lot about *training heart rate*. This refers to the heart rate, or pulse, necessary to achieve a proper degree of physical fitness. Achieving this training heart rate will have significant effects in terms of conditioning, and using it as a measurement offers a simple way to gauge the appropriate amount of exercise for each person.

The training heart rate is generally 80 to 85 percent of the heart rate a subject can achieve without collapse and is a function of age, body build, and conditioning. The *target heart rate* is the rate a person should reach given his height, weight, and age, for a given amount and duration of exercise. Most of the target heart rates that have been used have been based upon data derived from subjects who were performing "maximal exercise"; that is, they were exercised to the point of exhaustion; and they were often young subjects who did not represent the average population. Moreover, these "maximal predicted heart rates" determined from the data of exercise physiologists are just numbers, and striving for them may do harm to a subject who is pushed too hard. I have, therefore, had to derive my own figures and have done so by establishing exercise-tolerance standards which reflect the training, the physical fitness, and the capabilities of the average patient seen in a doctor's office.

TABLE 2
Training Heart Rates (Beats/Minute)

Age	Ordinary Subjects	Athletic Subjects
20–25	143	156
26–30	140	153
31–35	137	150
36–40	133	147
41–45	130	144
46–50	127	140
51–55	124	139
56–60	121	136
61–65	118	133
66–70	114	131

If you are interested in a simple way of estimating your own training heart rate, you will find a rule of thumb in Appendix C. Also, there are formulas for calculating the peak heart rate and the average heart rate from the maximal heart rate. But the best way of determining your training heart rate is to take an exercise test and have your doctor tell you.

It is important not to exceed the limits given, particularly for older persons; of course, for heart patients, the rate must be determined by your physician. In any case, regardless of the rate, exercise should be terminated if symptoms such as dizziness, weakness, nausea, chest pressure, or shortness of breath occur.

How to Find and Count Your Own Pulse

Obviously you must learn to count your own pulse (heart rate). This is really very easy to do. I have taught many people to do it in less than five minutes.

Place the fingertips of the right hand over the artery in the wrist (the dotted line in figure 1). You will quickly learn to recognize a rhythmic beat, and a little exploration will show you where it can be felt most easily. Just press lightly with your fingertips on this artery and you will feel a rhythmic pulsation.

Count out loud at first, so that when you time it with the second hand of your watch, your concentration will be on the pulse. You want to know the rate per minute, so you count for 15 seconds and multiply by 4. Count your resting pulse, and then count your pulse again *immediately* (within five to ten seconds) after the completion of exercise.

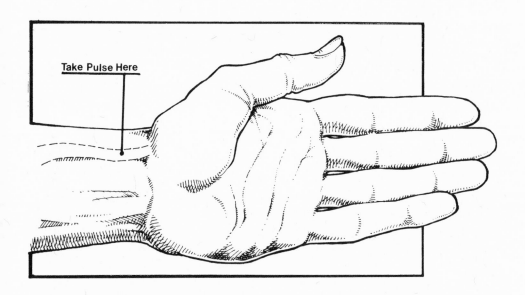

Figure 1. *Taking your pulse on your wrist.*

You can easily feel a strong pulse at the base of the neck, particularly after exertion. And many people have a good pulse in the temple. One word of caution: do *not* press high in the neck (see figure 2), because, as judo experts know, there is a very sensitive spot on the artery which can drop the blood pressure and produce fainting.

Heart rate can accelerate or decelerate quickly. Measurements have been made on the rate of change of heart rate at the onset of exercise. Two to three minutes of strenuous exercise will raise the heart rate to a top level. In all-out exercise, the peak is achieved after only 1½ minutes, as the amount of blood pumped increases immediately and stabilizes quickly. When you have completed your exercise, you must take your pulse *immediately* because, just as it can accelerate tremendously within one beat, it can slow down in a few seconds and you will miss the peak rate. Use a watch with a big sweep-second hand.

Your training heart rate is best determined by an exercise test, but if you take 80 to 85 percent of your top heart rate, it should fall somewhere between the average and athletic rates given in table 2, page 30. For the untrained, if it is lower, you are probably not exercising enough, and if it is higher, you are exceeding the safety level. For the average person, it usually lies between 120 and 130 per minute.

Training Heart Rate Slows as You Grow Fit

As training advances, some confusion may occur because two things take place: Your resting pulse is lower and your peak heart rate after a given amount of exercise slows as you become more fit. After some training, the heart rate after vigorous exercise slows to below 115 or 120 in five minutes and below 100 in ten minutes. Athletes will often reach their resting heart rates in this time. The less conditioned you are, the longer it will take you to reach your resting heart rate.

If you exert yourself to a maximum, your heart rate will accelerate to its top level. However, this is not dependent on training, but on age. You can be a superbly conditioned athlete and your maximum heart rate at a given age will be no higher than that of a sedentary subject. But the better your conditioning, the slower your *resting* heart rate and the slower your rate for a given amount of exercise. As you train, your heart can pump more with each stroke, so it does not have to pump as many times a minute.

M. H. started his exercise program at age forty-two because of an abnormal cardiogram and high blood pressure. His resting heart rate was 86, and after a ten-minute walk at two miles per hour, his peak rate was 143. His blood pressure at this point was 210/90. He was exhausted at first, but has faithfully pursued a vigorous walking discipline to this day. Now he is seventy-two, walks three miles in forty-two minutes up and down hills, and then goes for a swim. His resting pulse is 46 and his peak heart rate is

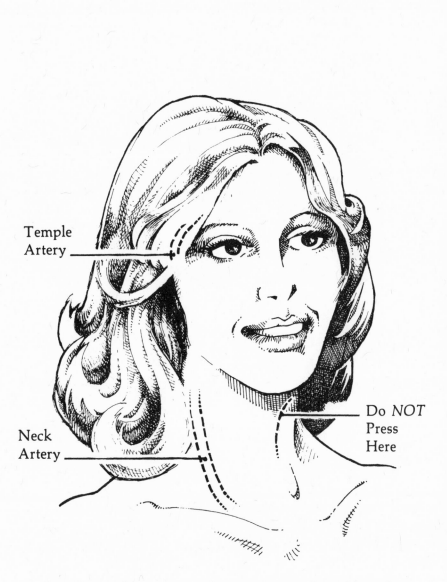

Temple Artery

Neck Artery

Do *NOT* Press Here

Figure 2. *Taking your pulse on your neck and temple.*

110 at a blood pressure of 140/60. His training heart rate has been lowered by his conditioning. He knows, from the time and distance he has covered, that his program is adequate, and he knows it from his sense of well-being.

The most striking change in heart rate occurs during the first few beats of exercise. The time it takes to empty the heart chambers decreases almost immediately regardless of the degree of the work load. In studies on tennis (see chapter 5) I have observed this immediate change in the first exchange of balls, and you can prove this by taking your own pulse. Obviously, this change must take place largely through the nervous system and release of adrenalin-like substances. In short, we are so geared that within one beat we can accelerate our heart rates and pump more blood. If there is excitement, the resting heart rate of even a marathon runner can exceed 100.

As you become more fit, your resting pulse will be lower, probably 60 or less, and you will be able to do the same amount of exercise at a lower peak rate. By measuring heart rate you can—

1. make sure you are exercising enough to achieve effective training;
2. stay within the 80 to 85 percent safety range;
3. follow your progress;
4. detect irregularities which should be reported to your physician for evaluation.

R. T. was a sixty-year-old man who had never been very athletic. His complaint was that he was always tired. He was a real-estate executive who spent most of the day on the telephone with his clients. At the end of the day, he dragged himself home, ate his dinner, and flopped in front of the television set. His wife loved sports and greatly enjoyed their paddle tennis court. But he was too tired to join in. At his wife's insistence, he came in for an examination. His health was excellent, despite his extremely poor conditioning. His blood pressure and blood sugar were normal; he was not low in thyroid or vitamins. On the treadmill, his resting pulse was 94, and at the lowest level, he got out of breath and his legs ached badly. He had to stop at 2½ minutes. At this point, his heart rate was 156, and after 8 minutes of rest, it was 112. He agreed to a progressive exercise program and began walking longer and longer distances at a faster and faster gait. In two months, his resting heart rate was 68 and his peak rate, just at the end of exercise, was 130. In the third month, he began a three-minute program of alternate running and walking. His resting heart rate was then 58 and his peak rate was 118. He had lost his fatigue, and everyone noticed his new enthusiasm and loss of irritability. And his wife is much happier because he plays paddle tennis with her and her friends.

Heart rate is used to measure a work load that is related to the maximal heart rate of the individual's age. At ages twenty to twenty-nine, it averages 180, but may exceed 200; at thirty to thirty-nine, it averages 170; at forty to forty-nine, it is 160; at fifty to fifty-nine, it is 150; and at sixty to sixty-nine, it averages 140. You can see that with every decade it declines approximately ten beats, or one beat per year. This varies with the individual, of course, and is best determined by exercise testing, but a handy rule of thumb is that it is 210 minus your age (see table in Appendix C).

Calories Measure the Amount of Work You Do

Energy is measured by work units, such as calories. The body gets its fuel from complex food substances—energy foods—which are broken down into carbon dioxide, water, and heat, measured in *large calories* (the amount of heat it takes to raise one kilo of water one degree centigrade). The number of calories burned per minute when you are at complete rest is your *basal metabolic rate*. Table 3 shows how you burn more calories as you increase your activity.

TABLE 3
Calorie Expenditure

Activity	Calories Burned Per Minute by 150-Pound Person
Bed rest	1.0
Walking (2½ mph on level ground)	3.6
Walking (4 mph on level ground)	5.8
Tennis (doubles)	7.1
Tennis (singles)	8.0
Cross-country running	10.6
Swimming (45 yards in 1 minute)	11.5

Calorie consumption, or energy requirements, has been determined for all conceivable types of activities. Playing singles tennis, for example, burns the same number of calories per minute as walking five miles per hour, cycling eleven miles per hour, swimming, splitting wood, shoveling snow, mowing the lawn, folk dancing, downhill skiing, or water skiing.

Singles tennis rates Number 1 in my book—it is a love match for your heart. It can be played by people of all ages and many conditions. It is relatively inexpensive and convenient, and its stop-and-go (Dash Training) quality is exactly what this doctor orders (if individual examination gives the green light). Swimming has been called the ideal exercise, but it is interesting to note that in swimming there is a ceiling to the heart rate, producing a lower maximal oxygen intake as compared to running sports. Vigorous ethnic folk dancing is excellent. Try it—after tennis, if you're not too pooped! Other good activities: lively table tennis, cross-country hiking, horseback riding, rowing, softball, and the like.

Eight to 10 calories per minute are required for running at five miles an hour, galloping on horseback, mountain climbing, ice hockey, snowshoeing, scuba diving, big-game hunting (including dragging the carcass), touch football, or paddleball. These sports are too strenuous for most middle-aged or older people. Ten to eleven or more calories are required for running 5½ miles per hour, cycling thirteen miles per hour, playing squash and handball, fencing, rope skipping, or vigorous basketball. These activities are for the young—or the athlete in top condition.

Doubles tennis consumes from five to seven calories per minute depending on the players, comparable to walking three miles per hour, cycling eight miles per hour, table tennis, golf only while carrying clubs on a hilly course, dancing, and most calisthenics. Doubles tennis is ideal for older persons, people with heart trouble, and, as my studies will show, can achieve the required heart rate for fitness. Walking is an absolute "must" if tennis is out of reach.

P. W. is now eighty. Before he started walking, he had had five proven heart attacks by the age of sixty-five! That should have given him a life expectancy of a few months. But he is still taking his daily walks with only a minimum of angina. He has worked out a unique way of relieving the monotony by walking through department stores. He knows his way around so well that he can maintain his pace while still seeing all the merchandise, as well as watching the women.

Playing golf while using a power cart ranks with playing billiards. It's equal to a nice brisk sit! But carrying your own clubs on a hilly course is beneficial. Besides, it's a great walk in a beautiful park with companionable people. Play golf this way when you aren't playing tennis.

Jogging is not on the recommended list if it means the stiff-legged trot which plays havoc with the human frame because of the jolts from landing on one's heels. It is included if it means a running stride taken on the toes, or running alternated with brisk walking.

Rope jumping is popular with people who are training for tennis. At ninety to one hundred jumps per minute, the work intensity is about equal to an eight-mile run.

TABLE 4
Activity Stairway

			Calories Burned per Minute
	Top Athletes Only	Running (5½ mph) Cycling (13 mph) Squash Rope Skipping Fencing Basketball Soccer	10–11
Minimum 30 minutes 3 times per week	*Too Strenuous for the Average Person*	Running (5 mph) Badminton Paddle Ball Handball Mountain Climbing Galloping on Horseback Touch Football Ice Hockey	8–10
	Ideal Level for Training and Heart Conditioning	Tennis (singles) Walking (5 mph) Cycling (11 mph) Swimming Skiing (downhill; water) Ice Skating Gymnastics Folk Dancing Rowing Digging Shoveling Snow Splitting Wood	7–8
	Best for Heart Patients and Those Over Age Fifty-five	Walking (3 mph) Tennis (doubles) Cycling (8 mph) Table Tennis Dancing Volleyball Calisthenics Golf (carrying clubs and climbing hills)	5–6
	Forget It	Walking (2 mph) Golf (using cart) Billiards	

3

There is some evidence that rope skipping may accomplish significant training in short periods of daily exercise. Dr. Kaare Rodahl, an associate of Dr. Astrand and head of the Work Physiology Department in Oslo, advocates rope jumping for all ages. He found that even five minutes a day could increase work capacity, but the individuals had to skip until they were out of breath. Other physical educators also advocate this form of exercise. It does tend to shape legs and hips, strengthen wrists and ankles, is an arm and leg exercise, and can be used in Dash Training when alternate rest periods are used. However, as rope skipping is very strenuous and its long-range effects are unknown, it must be used cautiously by people over forty. Moreover, it can cause deep warts on the soles of the feet and the feet can become chronically painful.

There are many nonsports activities that will provide conditioning and training. If you will count your pulse (see figure 1, page 31), you will be able to tell if the desired effects are being achieved. In the garden, you can hoe, dig, shovel, and rake. The care of a house involves sweeping, polishing, scrubbing, and ironing (3—6 calories). The carpenter can saw wood, sand, or nail (up to 8 calories). Painting; paperhanging; laying brick; using hand tools; assembling, repairing, or driving a heavy truck; plastering; pulling ropes; packing or stocking shelves (4 calories); waxing, washing, or moving furniture; carrying heavy objects; using pneumatic tools; chopping wood; shoveling snow; changing tires—all involve various degrees of work for the heart. And they will all qualify for adequate training *if* the heart rate is accelerated to the required level for the required time. But usually these activities are not performed on regular, continuing schedules, so the degree of fitness achieved will probably not be maintained.

PART II
Tennis and Other Racket Sports

Here be many other particular Recreations necessary for the knowledge and practice of our Husbandsman. . . . Health or action, are the Tenise or Baloone, the first being a pastime in close or open Country, striking a little round ball too or fro, either with the palme of the hand, or with Racket; the other a strong and moving sport in the open fields, with a great Ball of double Leather fild with Winde, and so driven too and fro with the strength of a man's Arme, arm'd in a Bracer of Wood, either of which actions must be learnt by the Eye and Practice, not by the Eare or Reading.

Country Contentments
or, the
Husbandsman's Recreations
Contayning the Wholesome
Experiences in which anyman ought
to Recreate himself, aftr the toyle
of more serious business.
Gervase M. Markham, 1649

Chapter 5.
Tennis Is Dash Training

Only recently have American medical publications been carrying articles extolling the exercise benefits of sports. The Germans recognized the relationship between gymnastics and medicine as far back as the 1930s, and sport in England was recommended for an increasingly industrialized society by the second decade of the twentieth century. The word *sport* comes from the English word "disport," meaning to frolic, gambol, and enjoy oneself in a relaxing pastime. It has been found that health can be substantially improved and maintained, provided one engages in the right kind of sport, virtually as a way of life. However, while young people pursue sports with enthusiasm and enjoyment, the aging adult, filled with the stresses of life, often abandons the very activity that would release tensions, provide an outlet for frustrations, stimulate muscles and circulatory system to relieve fatigue, and keep a person at the peak of his or her powers for the longest possible time. Alpine mountain climbers sometimes give their greatest performances in their eighties because of continuous training and because they know just how much to climb and how often to rest.

There are many sports that are joyful and that fulfill the training requirements. However, because of its present popularity, availability, and exercise value, I have picked tennis as the Dash Training sport ideal for our goals.

The current mass movement of people of all ages into jogging and running sports has been truly remarkable. Platform tennis, handball, racket ball, badminton, squash, volleyball, and paddleball are all booming. It is estimated that seven million persons are jogging, but the number playing racket sports is much larger (estimated at thirty-five million). The splash of the swimming pool is drowned by the *pock-pock* of the tennis ball, and homes with tennis courts are commanding ridiculous prices. Private golf clubs are adding tennis courts and, for the less affluent, there are over six thousand public courts being built each year. Some $550 million was spent in 1976 on tennis equipment—up one-third since 1974. New devotees are spending their weekends at tennis ranches for intensive instruction. "Hot tennis" is a new indoor-outdoor game for all ages. Originating in Korea, it spread to Japan and now the United States. It is equivalent to table tennis in exercise value, occupies only a small area, and can even be played sitting down. Lester Halpert, of the Los Angeles Recreation Department, is teaching tennis to patients confined to wheelchairs with only slight modifications of the rules! And the players all feel it has helped them tremendously, both physically and emotionally.

Who Can Engage in Running Sports?

Patients are besieging their physicians with questions: Am I too old? Is my heart strong enough? Should I switch from golf? Can I stop walking and play tennis? Should I play singles or doubles? How long can I play? How often? Is it all right for me to play on hot days, windy days, in the desert, in the mountains, at higher altitudes? Should I run hard after the ball?

Tennis today is king of the sports. And I think it and similar games are here to stay. The whack of rackets hitting balls is a joyful sound because achieving a proper level of physical fitness is rich in fun, exhilarating, and companionable, and promises health for the heart, young and old.

For those to whom being fit is a way of life, sports can be continued indefinitely, although periodic medical evaluation is required for safety. For those who take up sports late in life, conditioning is mandatory. The heart patient must have a medically supervised program. But there are very few who must be excluded from participating in sports.

Training Value of Tennis

The energy expenditure involved in playing singles and doubles tennis obviously depends on a number of factors: age, sex, weather, quality of player, competitive spirit, length of play, emotional makeup of the player, conditioning. Some play the game leisurely with many rest periods; others hardly stop between sets and may play almost continuously for hours. For some players, it is a mild recreation; for others, it is a grueling match. Therefore, no set of statistics will apply to a particular individual, and for the heart patient, a special study is required (this is true of any sport).

Heart Rate Studies

According to published studies, the *maximal* heart rate achieved in singles tennis is 179 beats per minute, while the *average* heart rate is 144. Doubles rates are often much lower. Another study of the heart rate in singles play found it to range from 132 to 151 beats per minute (average 143 beats a minute) for sixteen top 25-year-old tennis athletes in Czechoslovakia. There was a five-minute warm-up period, ten minutes of match play, and twenty-six minutes of recovery.

It was determined that 54 percent of the time, the players were running, and 46 percent of the time, they were walking, which is typical of a Dash Training exercise. The playing time was about equally divided with the less active periods. During play, the average number of strokes was 62. The resting heart rates of these players averaged about 60. During warm-up, the average pulse rose to around 125, and during ten minutes of play, to 143, never falling below this figure despite nonrallying intervals, until play was terminated. In the last few minutes, the rate fell to 90 and was still 10 beats above the starting pulse rate twenty-six minutes later.

Figure 3 (pp. 44-45) shows the results of a study I conducted of middle-aged men and women playing tennis. Singles were played by those aged fifty to sixty-four and doubles by those aged fifty to seventy-two as shown in A and B. Three of the players had had open-heart surgery and six had suffered heart attacks. They could not be distinguished from the others. The purpose was to observe middle-aged and older people since the studies previously published concerned only healthy young men. The ranges of the heart rates during the five-minute rest period, the five-minute rally, the thirty-minute play, and the five-minute recovery are shown in D. A sample of an actual recording is shown in C. A few players had irregularities of the heartbeat, mostly harmless skip-beats. One had a rapid, irregular rate called atrial fibrillation. It was found that he always took a drink or two before playing. When a subsequent test was made without the alcohol, the irregularity did not occur.

Figure 3. *Heart rate responses to tennis.*

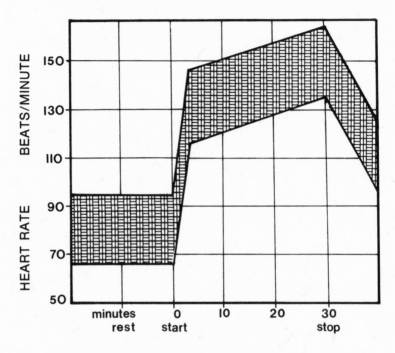

A. *Heart Rate during Singles*

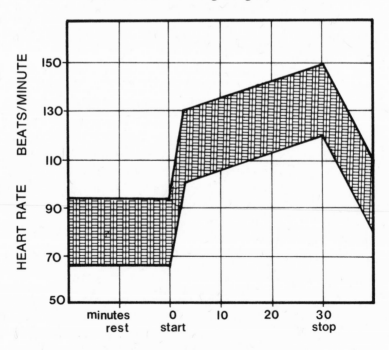

B. *Heart Rate during Doubles Play*

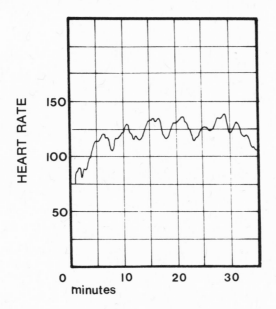

C. Sample Heart Rate Recording

	HEART RATE	BLOOD PRESSURE	B.P. × H.R. / 1000
5' REST	80 ± 14	105/80 - 165/114 Ave-126/86	10 ± 2
5' RALLY	118 ± 14	130/70 - 180/100 Ave-141/84	18 ± 4
30' PLAY	149 ± 11	135/75 - 200/95 Ave-152/84	23 ± 4
5' RECOVERY	107 ± 15	110/70 - 150/90 Ave-114/82	12 ± 3

D. Heart Rate and Blood Pressure Ranges

The average heart rate for singles was 139, varying by 11 beats up or down. The blood pressures averaged 152/84. The double product (see Appendix C) is the systolic pressure times the heart rate, and reflects the work of the heart better than the heart rate alone. As you can see, it doubles during play. This is a good training effect and does not put any strain on the player.

Doubles play shows an average heart rate of 120 and, of course, is less strenuous than singles. Note that as play continues, the heart rate gradually accelerates. This is an average response. Some players reach a plateau and stay there, but most do not. For older players who wish to continue playing for more than thirty minutes, it would be wise to count the pulse and not exceed the training heart rate.

Note that despite stop-and-go play, even in doubles, the heart rate stays elevated, varying only plus or minus about ten beats. Thus, tennis is a typical Dash Training sport, allowing older people to derive excellent training without undue strain or fatigue.

Playing Times for Games and Sets

In estimates I have made by stopwatch and hand computer, professional singles and doubles players average twenty-four minutes per set. Running play averaged nine minutes, while walking play, mostly serving, was eleven minutes. The ball was kept in play seven times over the net for an average point.

Nonprofessional singles games approach the professional time per set, averaging one minute and fifty-six seconds a game, and approximately twenty-one minutes a set. Doubles play for nonprofessionals is slower—about twenty-five minutes an average set. The ball is in play for amateur players about 4 points for doubles and only 3 times for singles. The longest nonprofessional exchange I recorded lasted thirty-eight seconds for 22 exchanges over the net.

These are approximations of considerable inaccuracy because of the obvious uncontrolled variations in players' skills and the number of games to a set, but it is possible to form some conclusions on the basis of them.

Most people need preliminary testing. All of our tennis subjects were first given a treadmill exercise test and their submaximal heart rates were determined in terms of duration of exercise and the work loads performed. Many had the sudden-exercise test as well as the heart watch (see chapter 12). They were classified according to age and sex, as well as presence of heart disease and physical capabilities. The results ran like this: Class I patients—the best—could attain work loads like those of young, healthy subjects. Class II patients did well, but in general were 10 percent below Class I. In Class III the attainable work loads were reduced by 30 percent. Class IV people were discouraged from playing tennis and were put on walking programs.

In people with histories of heart disease, age was a much greater factor. During the run-walk sequences of tennis, the fifty-year-olds reached peak heart rates of up to 165, but had averages of 140 at approximately 70 to 80 percent of the maximal heart rate. Ours are the only studies I know of that have been made of middle-aged and older players and of patients with heart disease.

The pulse rate remained remarkably constant during play and in most subjects varied only 5 to 10 beats. In contrast, an outstanding professional performing yoga showed tremendous variations: from 61 to 105 per

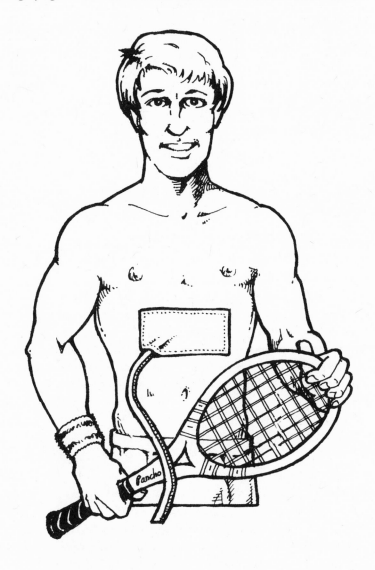

Figure 4. *Man is wearing heart watch during play to measure the heart rate.*

minute. The peaks were associated with expiration and the lows with inhalation, changing rapidly with each position. I would not recommend this isometric form of exercise for heart patients. This sort of rapid variation does not occur in tennis.

C. D. is a sixty-year-old man who has had a bypass operation. He first performed on the treadmill; then he was tested on run-walk sequences. Finally, the heart watch was applied during tennis, as in figure 4. His heart rates averaged the same for run-walk sequences and singles tennis and remained elevated at a constant level throughout both tests. Since playing tennis, he has lost his angina.

Dr. Edward H. Budd, president of The Travelers Insurance Companies, has pointed out the benefits from another racket sport—badminton. Studies by the Department of Physical Education at Baylor University showed that in a three-game singles match, for 20 of the 45 minutes of play each player had: 350 changes of direction, 400 swings at the shuttle, etc.—further supporting the value of sports training as both a health measure and fun.

Use Heart Rate to Check Progress

Measuring how close an individual comes to his maximal tolerable safe heart rate is a reliable index of the work performed and the amount of oxygen being burned. There are constant modifications when a sedentary person begins a training program. The resting heart rate slows, as does the peak heart rate, as the exercise progresses. For the normal person who has already been tested, reevaluation is usually not necessary, but for the heart patient, retesting at appropriate intervals is required in order to see that a sufficient work load is present and to guard against overload. If your heart is normal, you will find it useful to count your pulse and use the training heart rate formula (see Appendix C).

Singles Tennis Is "Heavy" Exercise

We have found that competitive singles tennis is in the heavy category of sports and the heart rates of middle-aged players reach 80 to 85 percent of the predicted maximal rate. The no-longer-young doubles players are in the moderate or even light categories, varying from 60 to 80 percent of their predicted maximum, depending on the vigor of play. In the coronary patients of Classes I and II, like the middle-aged normals, the heart rates vary between 125 and 165 and average 135 for singles and 125 for doubles.

Be sensible. Remember to play tennis wearing the proper clothing; know your tolerance under different weather conditions. Refrain from smoking, eating, drinking alcohol, coffee, or strong tea, especially either too hot or too cold, for about two hours before beginning to play. Spend ten minutes in a slowly increasing intensity of exercise during your rally period (before competition) and cool off for twenty to thirty minutes before taking a cold shower or a hot bath. Better still—avoid extreme temperatures, and if you must smoke, put off that cigarette.

What about tennis after fifty. . .or sixty? Many middle-aged and older people fear that it is too late for them to take up tennis because not only do they lack the physical stamina but they have lost the ability to coordinate their movements. Muscle strength does decline with age—but very little. In studies of neuromuscular coordination as a factor of aging, it has been found that the strength of the muscles of the arm and back do not change significantly from the ages of twenty to sixty-five, and reduced muscle strength—up to 19 percent—is found only in the seventy-to-eighty-year-olds. There is some loss of coordination, but the only significant decline occurs past the age of sixty-five, and the maximum for the oldest age (past eighty) is 30 percent. Therefore, even old people can maintain high levels of strength and agility if they exercise consistently, despite the known decline of maximal aerobic power and heart rate.

Intermittent exercise is the best form of exercise for people past middle age. Older individuals, despite their lessened abilities to use oxygen, can enjoy activities like tennis because of the short periods of exertion followed by periods of greatly reduced activity. Such activities do not build up large oxygen debts. The exercise involved is well within their capabilities. It also means that there is significant muscle training when high activity is alternated with rest.

As tennis involves both arm and leg work, there is more efficient training of the ability to use oxygen.

You Have to Be in Condition

Tennis is a special activity because it alternates short bursts of hard running with the relative inactivity of standing. Naturally, the young, vigorous person can usually play tennis without a second thought, although patients of all ages require exercise testing. The person who has played tennis all his or her life but is now in middle or older age still needs to be tested every year or two. The patient who has angina or who has recovered from a heart episode—be it an attack, a bypass operation, or the insertion of a pacemaker or a new valve—is a special situation (see chapter 6, "Safety in Sports"). But everyone needs conditioning, that is, steady exercise performed in a determined and persistent manner. There is nothing mysterious about it. You have to take the first step, increase gradually, and persist until the desired degree of physical fitness is attained. Then you have to continue the program to maintain your fitness. My mother is ninety-four, has always exercised vigorously, and is still taking her daily walks. When she was in her eighties, people used to call me and ask if I knew she was running down Wilshire Boulevard. In fact, one wag nick-named her, when she was eighty-five, the Westwood Flash.

Do you remember the story about the famous Roman gladiator, Milo? When he was a small boy and expressed the desire to be Rome's greatest athlete, he was advised by a wise man: "Every day carry a young calf three times around the coliseum." When the boy became a man and the calf grew into a bull, Milo became Rome's greatest gladiator. He didn't do this in twenty minutes a week.

When a proper degree of physical fitness is reached, singles or doubles tennis and similar sports may be played in safety, without undue strain or fatigue. Keeping active at the sport will insure your fitness and allow you to enjoy the exhilaration of competition, fun, and companionship, and the acquisition of a skill in a pleasant environment. And it avoids the tedium and boredom of walking on treadmills, performing calisthenics, or parti-cipating in exercise classes.

Advantages of Racket Sports

There are many advantages of racket sports:

1. They are pleasurable and cause much less tension and frus-tration than many other sports.
2. They are sociable and allow men and women to play together with equality.
3. They can be played at a level commensurate with the capabili-ties of the players, even those with heart disease or of advanc-ing age.
4. They relieve the tedium inherent in most exercises, which often leads to their abandonment.
5. They allow for warm-up by the nature of the preliminary ral-ly.
6. They raise the pulse rate to the training level required to achieve physical fitness.
7. The training level stays well in the safety area below the max-imal heart rate of the player.
8. They are intermittent and provide effective Dash Training, thus having a promising indication of protection against premature heart disease.
9. They involve arm and leg exercise, which induces a greater training effect while being physiologically less strenuous.
10. They can provide these benefits with thirty minutes of play at the training heart level three to four times a week.

"As to what our master has mentioned regarding weakness after exercise, the cause of this is its omission. If he resumes it gradually, little by little, he will find following it the strength and the vitality that should be found after all exercise that is carried out properly."

Maimonides, 1198

Chapter 6.
Safety in Sports

Death during a sport or other active physical exercise is a dramatic event, but despite the large number of sudden deaths each year (nearly half a million in the United States alone), only 2 percent occur from exertion. Seventy-five percent of sudden deaths occur at home, and 8 to 12 percent at work. Hippocrates described sudden death in 140 B.C., and in 1707 Lancisi was commissioned by the Pope to write *De Subitaneis Mortibus* ("On Sudden Death"). We are still studying the causes.

Under the auspices of the International Council of Sport and Physical Education, UNESCO, E. Jokl and J. T. McClellan published a monograph on cardiac deaths during exercise representing collected opinions on the subject up to 1971. There is no doubt that a well-trained athlete may still die of a heart attack. An apparently healthy young adult may have a defect of the coronary artery with which he was born. There may be rare infections of the heart muscle or even tumors of the heart. Blood vessels may have weak areas or heart valves may be diseased, causing them to be excessively narrowed or to leak badly. The heart may have blocks in its wiring system or beat rapidly and irregularly. There may be poor pumping of the blood or bleeding into the heart sac, the brain, or the lung. These conditions, some fatal, some not, can occur under a multitude of circumstances involving exertion not connected with sports—such as lifting a heavy object, moving furniture, chopping wood, gardening, and the like. Fortunately, death as a result of this kind of activity is very rare.

L. H. Opie has also written extensively on the subject in *Sudden Death and Sport*. Out of twenty-one deaths that he discussed, eighteen were caused by heart attack during or after athletic activity, and in this report, involved mostly playing rugby. There was one jogging and one yachting death. One death occurred during golf and two were associated with tennis. One of the tennis players was the club champion playing against a younger opponent. He was so determined to win that he played despite chest pain and died shortly after. The other tennis player also experienced pain but refused medical attention and died a few days later.

Interestingly, fifteen of the eighteen had chest pains or other warning symptoms, such as dizziness or excessive fatigue. The other three had brain and kidney disease. Moreover, thirteen of them were smokers, underscoring again the high risk of smoking. These symptoms and habits were known to their doctors and the patients before death, and many also had strong family histories of heart attacks.

Coronary Death Is Rare Among Marathon Runners

Dr. Thomas J. Bassler, a pathologist in Inglewood, California, has opened an unsettled controversy with several physician marathoners in South Africa and Canada, particularly Dr. Opie, because of Bassler's claim that no nonsmoking marathoner has died a coronary death proved by autopsy. Dr. Bassler implies that marathon runners are immune to death by heart attack. Dr. Opie cites three deaths which occurred in an annual South African fifty-two-mile race. All the patients had chest pain that they ignored. It would appear that, while even marathon runners can have coronary artery disease and die of it, such events are rare, lending support to the protective effect of vigorous exercise. This controversy is not likely to be settled soon because the necessary controls are difficult if not impossible to obtain; that is, to study thousands of people in similar age groups with the same risk factors, half of whom are marathoners and half of whom are not.

Dr. Bassler is president of the American Medical Joggers Association (AMJA), with centers in Toronto and Honolulu. Under its auspices, many heart patients have been trained to run up to twenty-five miles under the direction of a cardiologist. The statistics for proof of extended life are not yet available, although the recurrence rate of heart attack in this group is only 2 percent, as compared with the 25 to 35 percent of random groups. In this group, there have been no fatalities. However, trained cardiologist Dr. Terrence Kavanaugh, medical director of the Toronto Cardiac Rehabilitation Center, has achieved similar results. Dr. Joseph Mastropaolo, director of the Human Performance Laboratories of California State University, Long Beach, knew of only one death in eight years, and the cause was not ascertained. The risk of an untoward event in medically supervised exercise is estimated to be only one in six thousand hours. Some outstanding athletes have had significant valvular heart disease. Except in cases in which the heart muscle or its arteries was diseased, none of them suffered sudden death while engaging in sports. In nearly seven thousand cases, the percentage of collapse or death during sports activities was only 0.3 percent. In that 0.3 percent, autopsies showed serious cardiovascular disease.

Irregular Heart Rhythms Can Be Fatal

In sudden death, either the heart stops beating (cardiac arrest) or a disorganized quivering of the heart's muscle fibers occurs without an effective beat (fibrillation). Both, although fibrillation is more common, are responsive to resuscitation and electric shock. In a study of middle-aged Canadian businessmen, it was found that there was only one attack of fibrillation during 2,500 hours spent in a gymnasium.

When instantaneous death occurs, it is probably caused by such abnormal rhythms in over half of the cases, since autopsy shows only old disease of arteries. Patients with serious heart disease are undoubtedly subject to fatal arrhythmias, and if exercise precipitates too severe a stress, thus producing an inadequate oxygen supply to areas of heart muscle, sudden collapse is not surprising. The theme is still the same: It is not the sport which kills, it is the underlying disease.

Actually, a person prone to sudden cardiovascular death undergoes serious hazards even at rest or during minimal exertion. Such hazards are increased by anything that may suddenly elevate blood pressure, such as straining of the type that occurs with a difficult bowel movement, marked overdistension of the stomach, clots in the circulation, and so forth.

The emotional attitude of a player may also play a role. Excessive aggressiveness, conflicts, and the like are believed by some to precipitate fatal arrhythmias by provoking excessive stimulation of substances in the blood, like adrenalin, which overdrive the heart and make it vulnerable to rhythm disturbance. For the proper attitude, I recommend you read *The Inner Game of Tennis* by W. Timothy Gallwey.

Some deaths occur so suddenly and without warning that the coroner has to perform an autopsy to be sure the death was from natural causes. Such a study was done on 100 men in England. Acute psychologic stress was the immediate precipitating cause. Moderate physical activity, the time of day, or a recent meal, especially with alcohol, bore some relationship. But very severe exertion, the season of the year, the environmental temperature, chronic psychic stress, or the composition of the preceding meal had no relationship. The outstanding factor was acute emotional stress. Of course, the background was severe undiscovered coronary artery disease.

An amusing example of the effect of emotions on play occurred during a singles match between two middle-aged players. Both were strongly motivated by the desire to win. The match was nearly even for several games. Then, during a lull, one of them, who was wearing a contact lens after a cataract operation, began to blame his missed shots on his "floating" lens. Just then he overheard a spectator say, "What would he do if he knew the other guy had a glass eye?" What he did was to become so rattled he never won another game.

Others have found that more deaths are reported as occurring during competitive sports than during exercise training. Obviously, the emotion of trying to beat someone and being upset over losing is not going to contribute to your physical well-being. The sport should be pleasurable and played only for enjoyment.

High-Risk Subjects Are Readily Identified

In another Framingham, Massachusetts, study, 4,120 men were followed for sixteen years in an attempt to see if there were predictive factors which preceded sudden death. Of those who were studied, 234 (5.6 percent) died, and of those, 109 (2.6 percent) died suddenly. About 80 percent of those who died had no warning symptoms. But the high-risk patient could be identified early: high blood pressure, enlarged heart, abnormal electrocardiogram, heavy cigarette smoking, and the like. How to prevent fatalities? Alter the risk factors and stop, or at least slow, the advance of coronary disease by control of the risk factors.

Heart attacks are due to disease—not just the activity that preceded the attack. A recent review noted that nearly all sudden deaths can occur as a part of a general decline in health and be wrongly attributed to whatever activity the victim was pursuing at the time. Autopsies have disclosed that previously undiagnosed cardiovascular disease, diabetes, hypertension, and the like are nearly always present, so that the deceased would have been at risk in bed, let alone on the tennis court.

Proper Testing Is a Must!

Your physician can protect you if he or she is properly set up for exercise testing. Testing during strenuous activity requires special methods over and above standard testing. The following situation is not uncommon: A patient comes in complaining of chest pressure or pain whenever he makes a certain effort. Often he has been to other doctors who cannot explain his pain because his test results, even the exercise electrocardiogram, are normal. Again he is given the programed treadmill test, during which his speed of walking is increased from 1.7 to 4 miles per hour. He may or may not experience his pain, but the test is negative.

This is because the gradual warm-up has opened his accessory artery pathways and improved his circulation. If such a patient is rested and then goes immediately from rest to his target heart rate, he will experience pain and his electrocardiogram will often become abnormal. This is because his circulation has not had time to adjust to the sudden demand for oxygen.

Hidden Irregularities May Occur Only During Play

The monitoring of the patient during play has shown surprising abnormalities not revealed by the treadmill exercise test. We have seen evidence of dangerous arrhythmias as well as abnormal electrocardiographic changes. During play, there are emotions not present during routine exercise testing. If you are a heart patient and you get very excited, angry, or frustrated; if you hate to lose and battle hard to win, I advise you to get tested during play. In a recent experimental report (of the Cardiovascular Research Laboratory, Department of Nutrition, Harvard School of Public Health, Boston), Bernard Lown (noted for his basic studies on irregular heart beats and the use of electroshock) and his associates established that the nervous system contributed to fatal arrhythmias in a heart that has a poor blood supply.

Skip Beats

In the Tecumseh population study, over five thousand persons with skip beats (see chapter 13) of all kinds were followed for six years. It was found that the sudden death rate was very low and occurred in patients who had high blood pressure, high blood fats, and diabetes, and who were cigarette smokers. The conclusion is that skip beats require analysis. If they are found in conjunction with known coronary risk factors, they may indicate heart disease and be dangerous. But most people with skip beats do not have disease, and therefore there is no added risk. Again, a skilled cardiologist is needed to make the distinction. (See chapter 13, "Irregular Heartbeats.")

Remote Testing

Often it is necessary to test patients during their daily activities and away from the doctor's office. Many of the activities in which people engage are not simulated by office testing. There are several types of apparatus that are used for this type of remote analysis. One instrument that is quite complicated and expensive, called the Holter test, can record an electrocardiogram up to twenty-four hours on one continuous tape. When the patient brings back the tape, a special scanning instrument will sort out the abnormalities in these thousands of heartbeats. The patient keeps a diary, and a correlation is made between the day's events and the abnormalities seen on the tape strips. The patient records any unpleasant symptoms or sensations when they occur. The instrument will then show if there is any irregularitiy of the pulse or any evidence of impaired blood flow through the heart arteries at the time the symptoms were noted. These are indicated by the characteristic changes which a cardiologist can recognize in an electrocardiogram.

Besides the Holter test, there are several other devices used to record the heartbeat. The patient wears electrodes on the chest, and when he or she so desires, hooks up to a small detection device and turns on a portable tape recorder. Or the patient can place an appropriate instrument next to a telephone receiver, and the heart tracing is recorded in the doctor's office at the time the sympton is taking place. It can immediately be evaluated and instructions can be given to the patient via telephone.

Detecting Dangerous Irregularities

J. C. is an electronic engineer who enrolled in a jogging program. He had never been stress tested because, at the age of twenty-seven, he thought it was unnecessary. Every time he would run about a half-mile, he would become faint and dizzy, start sweating profusely, and have to stop. He would quickly take some sugar, and in fifteen minutes would recover except for a lingering sense of fatigue.

He saw a doctor, who told him he had hypoglycemia (low blood sugar), that popular, often-diagnosed but relatively uncommon condition, and put him on a high-protein diet. But eating before he ran only made him feel worse. He passed a treadmill test but complained of some pressure in his chest. So, he was sent for a heart artery X-ray. This proved to be normal. It was at this point that I saw him and attached our heart watch during his run. When his symptoms occurred, his heart rate suddenly accelerated to 220. We determined that this was due to a usually harmless arrhythmia called paroxysmal atrial tachycardia, which can be caused by stimulants and excitement. In this case, it proved to be the competition of running with his group that triggered his runaway rhythm, and it was easy to prevent with a medicine called propanolol.

The electrocardiogram may show a characteristic abnormality in over 60 percent of the patients with known angina who are totally unaware that there is anything wrong with them. It is possible to have a totally painless episode while driving a car! Smoking also induces frequent painless electrocardiographic abnormalities.

T. M. is an insurance vice president who had had two heart attacks by the age of fifty-three, but at sixty he had been entirely free of symptoms for seven years. When he decided to take up tennis, he underwent and passed a standard exercise test. But when monitored on the court he exhibited heart rates over 160 during mild play and many dangerous irregularities entirely unknown to the patient. Because of this, his arteries were X-rayed. He had severe three-vessel disease, which necessitated bypass surgery. Now he is playing tennis again and shows no abnormalities.

Obviously, there are patients for whom even the mildest activity is unsafe, and there are many others who should avoid strenuous exertion. Some of these cannot go 2 mph on a treadmill at zero grade without symptoms or abnormal signs—coronary patients with severe angina and three-vessel disease; patients with severe obstruction of a major valve; victims of severe arthritis; chronic alcoholics; patients with recent heart failure; patients with very large hearts, aneurysms, and the like, and lung patients with high pressure in the lung arteries. Naturally, these conditions must be determined by an expert.

Most irregularities are harmless. Many patients are needlessly concerned about thumping sensations in the chest, which constitute no risk whatsoever and occur in many normal people. Such sensations may be caused by nervous tension, coffee, tea, alcohol, or tobacco.

Alcohol and Tobacco Before Exercise Can Be Dangerous

The fact that acute and chronic alcoholism can cause sudden, unexpected death is well recognized. Often the victim was suffering from acute infectious disease. The lesson to be learned here is: Don't exercise if you have been drinking. And take seriously the warning that if you have a cold or mild flu, exercise may be harmful. Certain medications contraindicate strenuous exercise: muscle-relaxant drugs which markedly lower blood pressure and many sedatives, including antihistamines sold over the counter for colds. Heavy smoking before exercising can cause faintness. Inclement weather, either very hot or humid or very cold and windy days, impose marked stress. Wet clothing or too much clothing disturbs temperature regulation. Certainly no person with known heart disease should exercise under these conditions. Patients taking potassium-depleting drugs should have their blood levels checked. People have fainted or even had seizures when they have exerted severe effort at high altitudes or in hot, humid weather. And there is the "powerless attack" seen at the Mexico City Olympics, believed to be due to a temporary loss of muscle tone after an all-out effort.

Unrecognized Heart Attack without Exercise

In 9,509 healthy adults followed for five years, unrecognized heart attacks occurred in 3.6 per thousand as an annual average, while there were 5.3 recognized attacks per thousand. Half of the unrecognized ones were "silent"; that is, they caused no symptoms. In studies done in America, Finland, and Israel, for every heart attack that was recognized, there was at least one that was not.

Despite the extensive education efforts of our heart associations, many people are dying who could readily be saved by prompt attention. In California, a Rand study showed that it was taking an average of eight hours from the first indication of an attack to the time the patient reached the hospital. Most of the delay was due to ignorance or indecision.

In Los Angeles, paramedics answer most calls within five to ten minutes.

In the event that a person does experience a sudden heart attack, you stand a good chance of helping if you know what to do. If a person suddenly loses consciousness and has no pulse, strike him or her over the left part of the chest with a sharp blow. Often this starts the heartbeat. (Do this only if you have seen the person lose consciousness, and do it only once or twice.) If there is no response, start mouth-to-mouth resuscitation. Then follow these instructions:

Emergency Instructions
1. *Call fire department rescue squad.* Post the number for your local department near your telephone. A trained team will arrive in a very few minutes with oxygen and resuscitation equipment.
2. *Go to nearest emergency hospital.* A completely equipped hospital is preferable. Use the fastest transportation. Usually the rescue squad provides emergency transportation and oxygen.
3. *Call the doctor.* However, do not lose vital time trying to locate a doctor. Get the patient to an emergency hospital, which has life-saving equipment often not available to a doctor. In some heart stoppages, only electroshock can restart the heartbeat.
4. *Keep your telephone line open.* An emergency call cannot be answered if your line is busy.
5. *Learn mouth-to-mouth resuscitation.* The American Heart Association will supply you with illustrated instructions in this technique. Time is of the essence, and you may be the only link between life and death. If you know how—start CPR (cardiopulmonary resuscitation) immediately.

CARDIOPULMONARY RESUSCITATION
IN BASIC LIFE SUPPORT

Place Victim Flat On His Back On A Hard Surface

IF UNCONSCIOUS, OPEN AIRWAY

LIFT UP NECK
PUSH FOREHEAD BACK
CLEAR OUT MOUTH IF NECESSARY
OBSERVE FOR BREATHING

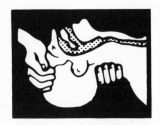

IF NOT BREATHING, BEGIN ARTIFICIAL BREATHING

4 QUICK FULL BREATHS

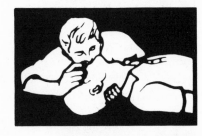

CHECK CAROTID PULSE

IF PULSE ABSENT, BEGIN ARTIFICIAL CIRCULATION

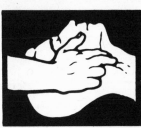

DEPRESS STERNUM 1½ TO 2"

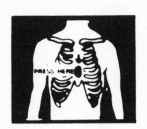

ONE RESCUER
15 compressions
rate 80 per min.
2 quick breaths

TWO RESCUERS
5 compressions
rate 60 per min.
1 breath

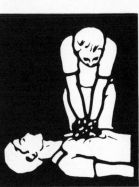

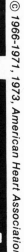

CONTINUE UNINTERRUPTED UNTIL ADVANCED LIFE SUPPORT IS AVAILABLE

Dr. J. Michael Criley and his associates at the Harbor General Hospital and the Cardiac Unit of the Groot Shur Hospital in South Africa have made a remarkable observation about patients whose hearts have stopped during the taking of coronary angiograms. Several patients who were urged to cough repeatedly were able to keep themselves from losing consciousness until their heart rhythms could be restored to normal. While it is a preliminary observation, it demonstrates that coughing can propel the blood like chest compression, and maybe in the future we will be teaching our heart patients how to resuscitate themselves. In the meantime it would be wise for everyone to learn and practice CPR on a manikin. Diagrammatic instructions are not enough. It has been shown that even physicians must view a teaching film, receive instruction, and practice on a manikin to resuscitate a patient properly. In many cities public programs are urging everyone to learn CPR.

Hazards of Tennis and Other Effort Sports

There is no doubt that there are certain hazards inherent in tennis and other sports. Some are physical effects, and others come from paraphernalia. In the early days of tennis, Louis X was said to have died from a chill caught during play. President Coolidge's son died from blood poisoning from a blister on his toe caused by an ill-fitting tennis shoe. Some people, as I do, wear contact lenses, and these offer opportunities for corneal injury. Wearing plastic sunglasses is particularly hazardous because if the frame breaks, the jagged pieces may pierce the eye.

After talking to optometrists, I concluded that the safest thing to do is to buy a pair of strong, steel-frame glasses, which will not shatter. Several times I have been struck in the eye by a fast ball, and my metal-frame glasses have saved me from injury. Rushing the net and being hit in the eye with the ball can result in serious contusion to the eye, with associated retinal detachment. If you have such an injury, be sure to have an eye examination immediately. It has been recommended that players wear protectors such as are used in handball, but I prefer the metal-framed sunglasses.

It is important to clear the court of stray balls. Many broken ankles, foot bone fractures, and wrist fractures from breaking falls with an outstretched hand have occurred because of tripping on a ball. Injury to the knees from cartilage tears, muscle-tendon ruptures of the legs, sprained ankles, heel bruises, and the like do occur.

The most common strain—to the elbow—is so frequent that *tennis elbow* has become a household term. There are many theories and conflicting reports about tennis elbow. An article in a British publication blamed it on metal rackets, while another report stated that fewer cases of tennis elbow occurred with metal rackets. Most professionals think a smaller grip and a lighter racket will reduce your chances of being injured this way.

A faulty stroke with excessive wrist and forearm torque, particularly during the serve and backhand, can result in the tendinitis around the head of the radius bone known as tennis elbow. I have found a valuable suggestion in the question-and-answer section of the *Journal of American Medical Association*. Before playing, or if the elbow feels strained, take the racket in hand and try to push it away from your body while restraining the movement in isometric fashion with the other hand. I have tried it and it works.

Even good players can get tennis elbow, and the pain can be so severe that it hurts to turn a doorknob. Armbands and wristbands, warming up with hot packs and cooling off with ice applications help, but not much. Tennis elbow can last a year. Most of the time, it is best to keep playing by warming up slowly and having a professional correct the faulty stroke that caused the problem. Injections of cortisonelike drugs are occasionally helpful, but carry such hazards as infection and weakening the tendon.

A word about diagnosis of tennis elbow. L. W. was a forty-two-year-old left-handed player who felt pain in his left elbow every time he played. He tried changing rackets, grip, and swing, went for X-rays and cortisone injections, but he still had increasing pain every time he played. He told me about his problem during his annual physical exam. The pain was so clearly related to effort that I put him on the treadmill and reproduced the pain and the characteristic electrocardiographic changes. What he was having was atypical angina—heart pain. Taking nitroglycerin before he played "cured" his "tennis elbow." Of course, he received full treatment for his coronary disease, and at present he has no problems.

Other Injuries

Such problems as clots in veins, neck sprains, back injuries, falls, and the like are bound to occur, and must be accepted as part of the game. Here, again, good physical conditioning will prevent or ameliorate most of these accidents. Those with joint problems should consult an orthopedist. There are people who develop migrainelike headaches after exertion, called effort migraine.

Most sprains are minor, and the best treatment is an ice pack and some aspirin. More severe injuries should be X-rayed. Women are particularly prone to injuries around the kneecap. A word about application of ice for minor injuries: It reduces swelling and pain, particularly if it is applied early; but the ice must be applied long enough to cool the deeper tissues, not just the skin—about twenty minutes. In more chronic injuries, heat can be effectively alternated with ice. If the pain becomes severe after initial improvement with ice, better call your orthopedist.

Warming Up Is Advocated

Warming up is particularly important for patients with heart disease, as it allows time for circulatory adaptation. But all persons should start exercise gradually, as this enables better utilization of all bodily systems, making injury less likely. In tennis, this is usually accomplished by the pregame rally. For the sake of the skeletal muscles as well as the heart muscle, allow at least ten minutes of warm-up before sudden effort.

Nitroglycerin Is Like Warm-Up

It has been found that persons with angina can perform much greater work loads if they take prophylactic nitroglycerin. The patient who would normally develop angina at a certain stage of exercise after warm-up can go to a higher stage without angina and without electrocardiographic changes. Therefore, it is always wise for a patient with angina to take nitroglycerin before any exercise. And there are times during play when it should be taken again. One friend with whom I play never gets angina except when the competition is keen and it is his turn to serve. He has learned that if he takes nitroglycerin at this point, he can avoid chest pain.

PART III
Exercise and the Heart Patient

The wise, for cure, on exercise depend;
God never made his work for man to mend.
                                John Dryden, 1669

Chapter 7.
Coronary-Risk Factors

Many people don't understand why so many tests need to be done during checkups. "I just came in to get my blood pressure taken," they say, "and they took all my blood, gave me X-rays and electrocardiograms. Who needs it?" Well, believe me, *you* need it. There are 450,000 sudden deaths every year, largely due to clinically detectable coronary disease. The American Heart Association has recommended that a physician not prescribe an exercise training program without first testing to see how much exercise the person can tolerate. Many heart associations, like that of Tennessee, have gone on record: "Any well person over thirty-five years old and persons of any age at risk or with disease predisposing to coronary artery disease should have an annual exercise test."

Admitting that our knowledge is incomplete, but insisting that we certainly know enough to institute effective measures, most heart associations agree that sex, age, high blood pressure, high blood fats, tobacco, and diabetes rank high among the factors producing disease. The National Heart and Lung Institute has been funding research proposals since 1971.

The chances of developing serious or fatal heart attack by age sixty-five are 37 percent for a man and 18 percent for a woman. Evidence has been accumulated for what are believed to be the known causes of coronary disease. The major coronary-risk factors are heredity, sex, and age. In order of their probable importance, the other principal factors are hypertension; tobacco; diabetes; lack of exercise; high blood fats (which include cholesterol and triglycerides); gout; and obesity. The roles of chronic tension and the so-called Type A personality (see page 79) and cholesterol, are still controversial. I will comment on each of these, but only as they relate to exercise, since each in itself has been extensively reviewed in the popular press.

Controlled Population Studies

In 1948, highly respected studies were begun in Framingham, Massachusetts, largely through the efforts of Thomas R. Dawber, who decided it would be valuable to observe cardiovascular disease in a general population sample. After over two decades of research into how such diseases begin and end and what factors make certain individuals vulnerable, a recent summary has been published in the *American Journal of Cardiology*.

These studies emphasize that coronary artery disease can attack without warning; sudden death may be its only sympton (a study by J. T. Doyle reveals that 25 percent of victims struck without warning die suddenly). Because such individuals can be identified *before* tragedy occurs, the chain of events leading to this can largely be prevented. The search for coronary-risk factors determines the kind of tests the doctor makes in evaluating your state of health during an annual physical examination: history as to cigarette smoking, events in your family, measurement of your blood pressure, tests of your blood sugar and cholesterol, and your electrocardiogram at rest and after exercise. Periodic testing can identify a very high percentage of asymptomatic disease. There are millions of people in the United States with diabetes and high blood pressure, half of whom don't even suspect that these killers are present but could find out through such testing.

Such sudden deaths represent medical failures, because they result from conditions that should have been detected years ago. In the Framingham community, where the population was unusually aware of heart disease, one in four heart attacks went unrecognized, half being "silent" and half so atypical that neither the patients nor their physicians even thought of the diagnosis. One in five of the deaths was sudden; the first and last event. Two-thirds of the deaths occurred without any medical care.

Coronary-risk factors are known defects for which a doctor can easily test, and their detection and control can greatly affect the life expectancy of the patient. In two decades of the Framingham study, the death rate from coronary disease was very low among individuals who had no risk factors and rose progressively to very high figures as each risk factor was added. Of course, proper medical evaluation of a person may show that the risk factor is very low and thus be reassuring. This is particularly true for people who are needlessly alarmed over the presence of a single risk factor, such as a moderately elevated cholesterol level.

Can Young People Die of Heart Attack?

Many people think coronary disease is a disease of old age. But in fact it is present among people of nearly all ages past the age of twenty. Among 300 United States soldiers killed in action in Korea, significant coronary disease was found in 77 percent, and 15 percent had more than 50 percent obstruction of a major artery. F. S. Pettyjohn and R. R. McKeekin report similar findings in Vietnam casualities and in casualty autopsies conducted by the Armed Forces Institute of Pathology, where 89 percent had coronary artery disease. The presence of coronary-risk factors in men under forty is worldwide, according to M. A. Dolder and M. F. Oliver, although the number varies and the importance of each factor varies in different nations. For example, cholesterol levels were relatively low in Australia, but cigarette smoking was high everywhere. The highest rates of coronary disease are in Finland and the United States, with lower rates in Greece, Japan, and Yugoslavia, and the lowest rates of all in Nigeria. But in all countries, the implications are the same: Even young men do not escape heart attacks when known health principles are violated.

While age is a principal determining factor, many old persons escape atherosclerosis, the disease we're talking about. Genetic factors are important, but the disease often ignores even such influences through little-understood immune mechanisms natural to the body. People are not necessarily doomed by heredity.

High Blood Pressure

The worst risk factor is high blood pressure, a disease that in the vast majority of cases is easily controlled. It is estimated that there are twenty-three million such persons in the United States today. Only half know it and half of these are untreated. Elevated blood pressure greatly accelerates disease of the blood vessels. The upper pressure (the systolic) is just as important as a predictor of trouble, or maybe more so, than the lower (diastolic). My patients are always asking about cholesterol, but they don't seem to attach nearly as much importance to blood pressure. The Framingham study revealed that high cholesterol has relatively little influence when the blood pressure is low. There are 1,700,000 strokes per year in the United States. The chief cause is high blood pressure. Among the nondrug methods of controlling high blood pressure, exercise and weight reduction are the most important.

The Joint National Committee on Detection, Evaluation and Treatment of High Blood Pressure of the U.S. Department of Health has recommended that all persons with a diastolic pressure of 105 millimeters of mercury pressure or higher be treated. If the diastolic pressure is between 90—104, treatment should be individualized. Pressures should be taken while the subject is sitting comfortably and repeated several times to obtain an average. If the pressures are borderline, such as 140/90 to 160/95, they need to be rechecked every three months.

Everyone should be checked once a year. For those who take their own blood pressures, it is important to understand that the diastolic pressure is measured at the *disappearance* of sound. While systolic (see Appendix B) pressure is also important, the benefits of treatment are not so clearcut, and a physician must judge when special tests are necessary to define the cause of the elevated pressure. Most patients with persistent elevations will require the use of one or more antihypertensive drugs administered under a life care program.

Cholesterol

The machinery of our modern technology has replaced our muscles, so that the too-rich food we eat is not offset by a necessary expenditure of energy, and this results, of course, in overweight. Hence, lack of exercise appears to be an important contribution to the development of hardening of the arteries. While the relation of diet to elevated cholesterol levels in the general population is far from clear, an energy balance unable to cope with the overload of fat may be the deciding factor. In my own practice, I find a very inconstant relation between cholesterol level and coronary heart disease. I once prepared a list of over two hundred individuals matched as to age, sex, and so forth. Half had had heart attacks and half were healthy, according to careful evaluation. My colleagues were unable to distinguish which group had had the heart attacks by reading their cholesterol counts, even though many of the patients had values recorded over ten to twenty years. It should be understood that "normal" cholesterol levels rise with age and vary in different regions of the United States, other countries, and other populations. A former rule of thumb was that the cholesterol level should be 200 plus your age. But no firm figures can be used as a guide particularly since laboratories make frequent errors and differ in their standards. Leading investigators now think that the uppermost level should be 240 mg by the Abell-Kendall standard. Irving S. Wright reports that in Japan, common levels of cholesterol are as low as 170 to 200, perhaps because of the vastly different dietary habits there. The Japanese in America have American cholesterol levels.

The relationship between cholesterol and heart disease is still being debated. After sixty-four years of research, many thoughtful doctors do not accept the proposition that high cholesterol causes heart attacks any more than high blood sugar causes diabetes. It may be more logical to think of high cholesterol as the *result* of artery disease and not the cause. Dr. William R. Castelli, director of laboratories of the Framingham Heart Studies, has emphasized that a high *total* cholesterol count is not a reliable indicator because there are several kinds of cholesterol. Cholesterol in the blood stream is attached to substances called lipoproteins. The alpha type of cholesterol (high-density lipids, or HDL) actually helps transport cholesterol out of the blood. The University of Oslo has found that if HDL is too low, more heart disease occurs, and a report from Hawaii on Japanese men has substantiated this finding. The beta cholesterol (low-density lipids, or LDL) contained in fatty foods is the one connected with increased arterial disease. If this cholesterol hypothesis stands up, these two substances— and probably others—will have to be separated. Parenthetically, exercise *raises* HDL and *lowers* LDL. It should also be pointed out that this separation of cholesterollike proteins into those which are disease producing and those which are protective is a new observation. Previous work on total cholesterol now loses much of its significance since it was not known how much of it was "good" or "bad." And it is not clear what foods may finally be implicated.

Dr. Mark D. Altschule, one of our most respected medical writers, says: "If all you want to know is whether so many of your favorite foods, such as eggs, that contain cholesterol *increase* your risk of heart disease, *they do not!* If you want to know whether those TV ads for 'substitute' foods that loudly proclaim 'no cholesterol, no animal fat' are a lot of pseudoscientific nonsense, *they are!*"

These convictions do not apply to those with a strong family trait of very high cholesterol counts and a strong family history of early heart attack. This is a special group, and modern doctors begin at the pediatric level to find these patients. But they are not to be confused with the general population. Dr. Risteard Mulcahy, director, Cardiac Department and Coronary Heart Disease Research Unit, St. Vincent's Hospital, Dublin, has found that lowering cholesterol may not importantly affect longevity.

Worldwide population studies have shown that people who were fed normal and high-fat diets exhibited no differences in the number of heart attacks they had. All these statistics have produced no conclusive results except to say that coronary disease is more frequent if the cholesterol is elevated. Much work is now being done with the origin of disease in the cells of the artery itself. Here is where the cholesterol forms and gets into the bloodstream. According to Dr. Earl P. Bendit, chairman of the Department of Pathology of the University of Washington School of Medicine in Seattle, if a cell is injured by a poison like tobacco, it makes fat instead of protein. From this may develop the "plaque" which slowly obstructs the passageway of the artery and blocks the flow of blood (see figure 8, page 134).

H. M. Whyte reports on a study where men aged thirty-five were divided into two groups: Half were kept on low-cholesterol diets and half ate as they pleased. When they were fifty-five, twenty years later, there were only 6 percent fewer strokes and heart attacks in the low-cholesterol group. This means that for 94 percent, the program was without benefit, and 8 percent had heart attacks within twenty years despite low cholesterol. The benefit of such a program is less for women and much less for those who start at an older age. Moreover, there is no consistent progression of disease in those with elevated cholesterol levels, nor are all populations equally affected. The Masai eat large quantities of saturated fats but have a low frequency of heart attack, possibly because of their high level of physical exercise.

From birth, the population of Slieve Laugher, Ireland, has an exceedingly high consumption of animal fats because they are dairy farmers. And the most common cause of death among males is cardiovascular disease, according to Albert and J. G. Casey. But they live longer than their wives by 2.5 years (over age seventy-six) and 8 years longer than United States males when this study was reported in 1969. Much more needs to be learned before cause and effect become clear. If high-cholesterol levels do carry a risk, it seems likely that this is over a long period of time, so a corrective program should start at a young age.

Cholesterol in Our Food

Peter N. Herbert (a National Heart Institute Fellow and Investigator) reports that present investigations at the National Heart Institute of Health are radically changing our ideas of diet in relation to cholesterol. An amazing finding is that eggs can be eaten as desired with little effect on the blood cholesterol if they are not of the dry-powdered variety (many processed foods contain substances that can damage blood vessels). In a study by Bruce E. McDonald and associates from the Department of Foods and Nutrition at the University of Manitoba, Winnipeg, up to 6 eggs a day for 2–3 months were eaten by healthy young men (up to 1500 mg per day). While the cholesterol rose, the values never exceeded normal limits. You may ask how, after all these years of preaching against eggs, we can now tell you they're all right. Isn't the yolk of the egg pure cholesterol? It now appears likely that if there is in fact a food culprit, it is the low density lipoproteins, the fat derived chiefly from fatty meats and milk products. In fact, cholesterol itself is normally found in all body cells; and if the cell does not contain any, it will die. If it does not get enough from the blood, it will make it itself. When eggs without saturated fats like that in sausage and bacon were fed to patients, the extra cholesterol went into the liver and was sent out as bile into the gut. The level of cholesterol in the blood did not rise. In order to reduce the cholesterol blood level by changing the diet, you have to sharply limit meat (even the lean part contains lipoprotein), cheese, the skin of fowl, and processed foods. Most of all, you have to limit calories to achieve a lean body weight. An interesting observation has come out of India: Eating onions, cooked or raw, with a fatty meal prevents a rise in cholesterol, apparently by blocking fat metabolism. The significance of this is as yet untested.

A 1976 Tecumseh population study on dietary habits and fat in the blood concluded that the amount of fat, sugar, or alcohol consumed is not as important as how fat you are. An important point is that when the dietary habits of population groups are studied, there may be a correlation between cholesterol and heart disease, but when applied to the individual, the relationship often does not hold up.

There are probably thirty million Americans who cannot drink milk without developing symptoms like irritable colon, diarrhea, abdominal pains, excess gas, and the like. Contrary to dairy product advertising, many people not only outgrow their "need" for milk, but they don't have a specific substance in their bowel, "lactase," to digest it, says T. M. Bayless of Johns Hopkins University. Milk has even been named as a cause of heart disease. Shellfish are probably all right because the substance in them is another sterol, not cholesterol.

It is still generally recommended that unsaturated fats like safflower and corn oil be used for cooking and for salads, but some think they add to heart disease and are even linked with cancer. When the damaged artery cell starts making fat, the type is *unsaturated!* Mixes prepared with coconut oil are to be avoided. As pointed out by Drs. Katherine Clark and Frank Marcus in a letter to *Circulation* magazine in 1976, some of the health-food cereals like Granola contain large amounts of unsaturated fats like coconut oil. A half-cup of a Granola cereal contains 9.5 grams of saturated fat—or the total amount of saturated fat allowed per day in a healthy diet. Such unlabeled foods can completely defeat a dietary program aimed at restricting saturated fat. A liquid or semiliquid oil is usually unsaturated; when solid, it is "hydrogenated," that is, it becomes saturated and loses its cholesterol-lowering properties. Chocolate is still on the no-no list, I'm sorry to say.

Cholesterol has been in and out since 1913 when Nikolai Anitschkow first fed high-fat diets to the vegetarian rabbit and produced artery disease. As a medical student, I used to spend my summers working for the great biochemist Meyer Bodansky, who wrote the standard textbook of that time. I removed tiny thyroid glands from baby rats and rabbits and fed them various diets in order to study cholesterol and artery disease. This was my first participation in scientific research. Our researches were as inconclusive as much of the evidence today. I think we do know that *how much you eat* is much more important than *what you eat*. In any case, if you want to find out how diet affects you in blood tests, you don't have to go on a lengthy program. Two to three weeks will usually tell the story.

I think all this controversy and inconsistency will some day be explained by new methods of testing for the "good" and "bad" types of cholesterol. If one harms and another protects—and we are just finding all this out—previous studies which confused the two are nearly worthless. The terms *HDL* and *LDL* will soon become as familiar as *cholesterol*, and you will be much further along in your quest for better health through diet.

Arguments FOR and AGAINST the Cholesterol Hypothesis

FOR

1. Excess cholesterol in the form of "Chylomicrons" deposits in injured artery lining to form "plaques."

2. The higher the excess of cholesterol from fat-rich meals, the more the deposit in the arteries.

3. Wherever the cholesterol in the blood is high, population studies show a high incidence of atherosclerosis (disease of arteries).

4. Where the cholesterol is low, there is very little chance of a heart attack.

AGAINST

1. Dr. Earl P. Bendit has shown that the injured cell stops making protein; it starts to make cholesterol which gets into blood stream.

2. Every cell in the body will die if it does not have cholesterol. If it receives a lot *externally*, it makes little; if none, it makes a lot.

3. There are groups with very high cholesterol counts and very little chance of a heart attack. Both HDL and LDL must be measured.

4. Many people with a "normal" cholesterol level have heart attacks. It is high in many animals and fishes—500 mg. in a salmon.

5. Population studies show that those who eat fat-rich diets have much more artery disease than those who eat fat-poor diets.

5. These studies have not distinguished between low-cholesterol and low-calorie diets causing weight loss. Many feeding experiments show *no difference* in death or disease rate in the two groups. Even where the heart death rate seems to be lower, the cancer rate is higher. Where alpha cholesterol is low, there is more disease. Stroke is not related to cholesterol level or even weight.

6. Animals fed high cholesterol foods develop artery disease like humans.

6. Such diets contain processed foods that form substances damaging to arteries and not present in natural foods.

7. Processed foods form substances that can damage arteries.

7. Studies on animals and humans where severe stresses are induced or present show a lower degree of heart disease.

8. Type A behavior pattern causes high cholesterol and diseased arteries.

8. The cholesterol attitude is largely American. The British Heart Association has not endorsed it. Drugs which lower it have not reduced rate of heart attack.

You Don't Have to Be Fat

The best way to lower cholesterol is to lose weight. I know all the arguments, but if you want to stay lean, you can either be hungry and inactive, or if you want to eat what you wish, you must be very active. If you cover 3 miles a day at a brisk walk, you will burn 8000 calories in a month. This is 2 pounds of body fat. An afternoon of tennis will burn approximately 1000 to 1200 calories; three times a week, 3600 calories. In a year of such activity: about 45 pounds! Losing weight by exercise also prevents sagging, because what is burned this way is all fat and spare tissue.

If you want to do your own weight-loss figuring, look at the calories burned per minute on the Activity Stairway on table 4 on page 37. Multiply the calories burned by the minutes exercised. Then multiply by 7 for the week's loss. Since 4000 calories equals one pound of body weight, divide your answer into 4000 to find the number of pounds you would lose in a week.

The danger of obesity leading to disease of the arteries in middle or later life has not been stressed enough. While I have indicated that the issue of cholesterol in the diet is still controversial, I want to emphasize that overweight leads to high blood pressure, diabetes, elevated blood fats, and the subsequent heart attack or stroke and sudden death. The coronary epidemic began when our young people started to eat too much and exercise too little. It is estimated that over 15 percent of our teenagers are fat. There is a 90 percent chance that by the time they reach the age of thirty, they will be obese—25 to 30 percent overweight. And most of them are sedentary. The coronary epidemic will not be controlled until our young people learn to stay lean and vigorous, which will also contribute to increased longevity.

A word about diets. Every magazine carries a new one. Every "fat doctor" has a new gimmick. Some claim you can pound or rub the fat off by "breaking it up." And of course there are the pills and shots that "alter metabolism." The most popular, which received pseudoscientific support, is the one based on the "pituitary hormone," chorionic gonadotropin. A recent critical diet study, in which neither the patient nor the shot-giver knew whether the shot was water or the hormone, showed that there was absolutely no difference in effect. The weight loss was due only to the 500-calorie restriction imposed on the subjects. The fat doctor, who usually insists on payment in advance, has the subject come in every day for a shot, get on the scale, and answer questions about his diet. And the dieter does lose weight, but since nothing has been learned about calorie values, nor have eating habits been changed, the weight is quickly regained.

Dr. Frederick J. Stare, professor of nutrition, Harvard School of Public Health, and his co-author, Dr. Elizabeth M. Whelan, were asked to rate the ten top diets in vogue today.

In their book *Panic in the Pantry* they say that the Atkins Diet, low in carbohydrates and high in fat, is boring and nauseating. The lack of sugars, our "brain food," causes headache and fatigue and raises the level of uric acid. The high amount of fats has been condemned by the American Medical Association's Council on Nutrition as dangerous to the heart. Similar defects are found in the Stillman Diet which is too low in carbohydrates, nonsensical in terms of defying the laws of thermodynamics, deficient in vitamins and minerals, etc.

The Last Chance Diet of Dr. Robert Linn, an osteopath, is really a starvation diet suitable only under strict medical supervision or in a hospital. It leads to a loss of glycogen (a source of stored sugar) in the liver and a loss of potassium and sodium. The resulting acidosis leads to high blood levels of uric acid which may precipitate gout. Dr. Frank's No Aging Diet is "a massive network of scientific gobbledygook." The HCG Diet (chorionic gonadotropin shots) exposes the subject to unknown long-term effects and relies on 500 calories a day for weight reduction.

Now making daily headlines, the Pritikin Diet claims to cure heart disease with a fat-restricted program. But Pritikin allows only 10 percent of the daily caloric intake to be fat—"an extremism that is unrealistic," says Dr. Stare. "You cannot undo the effects of years of overeating by restricting fat intake for one or two months (and it is unlikely that you would stick with this diet longer than that)."

Dr. Reuben's Save Your Life Diet is based on the use of high fiber foods. Although bran and other fiber foods do seem to benefit the colon, there is no evidence that they prevent heart disease or aid longevity. The Crenshaw Super Diet promotes kelp and lecithin, but in the opinion of Stare and Whelan, with "absolutely no scientific basis." The Macrobiotic Diet is called a "mixture of occultism, mysticism, religion and dietary extremism, promising to cure all illness." The diet is so deficient that some young Americans have actually starved to death. The Jolliffe Prudent Diet has many versions, but the principle of eating a variety of foods in moderation is endorsed by most physicians.

The latest fad is the "predigested protein" liquid mixture supposed to make the subject lose fat and "spare protein." As was pointed out by Dr. George V. Mann of Vanderbilt University, there is little or no evidence that only fat will be burned on such a diet. He also points out that the role of exercise in getting rid of excess fat was ignored: those who undertake physical training tend to become lean and muscular even with a free intake of food. The safety of such a program is also in question. Look at the diets that have come and gone in the last few years: Atkins, the Zen Macrobiotic, Adelle Davis, Reuben, Taller, Franks, and Stillman. But it's the latest one that is always the answer. Dr. Stare says, "The road to Utopia is paved with fad diets."

Food Additives

Everyone is now afraid of *food additives*, so much so that even beneficial substances are suspect. Dr. Thomas H. Jukes of the Division of Medical Physics, University of California, Berkeley, has pointed out that one would hesitate to drink a beverage containing trimethyl xanthine and chlorogenic acid. What is it? It's coffee. And he indicates that using "natural" foods can also be unsafe: sassafras root and honey have been found to contain substances that are carcinogenic, that is, can lead to cancer. The FDA lists 670 substances as food additives. The "Delaney Clause" of the Food Additives Amendment of the Federal Food, Drug And Cosmetics Act states that no additive can be deemed safe if it is found to induce cancer in man or animals. But, of course, the FDA cannot affect such substances found naturally in foods. The leading food additive is sugar, because it prevents spoilage in foods such as jams and jellies. The organic and health food movements have become so emotional about sugar that the senate committee on nutrition cut the *recommended* U.S. intake by 40 percent. Dr. Jukes points out that the committee simultaneously suggested that the proportion of carbohydrates in the diet be increased.

Salt is another common food additive. It can cause high blood pressure, and we all probably eat too much of it. As to vitamins and minerals, Dr. Jukes believes that the 10 necessary vitamins and essential minerals could be added to foods at a cost of one dollar per person per year. Synthetic vitamins, contrary to popular dogma, are either identical to natural vitamins, or, in some instances such as folic acid, are more effective. He does not share Dr. Ben Feingold's opinion that synthetic chemicals are villains or that artificial food colors cause behavioral disturbances in children. Jukes believes that the necessary research for such conclusions was never fully carried out.

Jukes concludes that "the most injurious of all food additives is the additional food that is eaten after the calorie needs have been satisfied. Overconsumption of food leads to obesity, which is a far greater danger to health than any of the food additives whose safety is now being questioned."

Megavitamins Can Do Harm

Some of the most gifted and otherwise intelligent people I know stuff themselves every day with handfuls of vitamins and other food supplements with the belief that they feel better, are more active sexually, and are protecting themselves from disease. They also believe that these practices are free of risk, and when advised otherwise by their physicians, they say, "Doctors don't know anything about nutrition!" Well, here is what Dr. Victor Herbert, chief of the nutrition laboratory at the Bronx Veterans Administration hospital, has to say: "Megavitamin therapy is largely nutritional nonsense."

Megavitamin dosages are far above the known requirements for vitamins even in the face of real deficiencies. For example, 10 mg of vitamin C taken daily will cure scurvy. This is a disease that British sailors used to get during long voyages at sea without fresh fruits or vegetables. Later it was discovered that the bleeding of the gums, muscular pains, etc. of this deficiency state could be prevented by small amounts of lime juice; that's how the British tar got to be known as a "limey." If there is any foundation for the use of vitamin C in colds, 200 mg is more than adequate. Actually, carefully controlled studies have been inconclusive, although there may yet prove to be some merit to vitamin C. More important, can these large doses do harm? Excess amounts of vitamin A can cause loss of appetite, retard the growth of children, cause the skin to dry and crack, enlarge the spleen and liver, produce loss of hair, joint pains, irritability and headache due to rise of pressure in the brain that may be confused with brain tumor. It also destroys vitamin B^{12}. Large doses of the B vitamins have caused liver damage in rats; folic acid can precipitate convulsions in epileptic patients. Nicotinic acid (of the vitamin B complex) in addition to flushing, can cause liver damage, rashes, and ulcers. Vitamin D can produce nausea, weight loss, bowel and urine disturbances, calcium deposits, high blood pressure, anemia, kidney failure, and even death.

Vitamin E has become the favorite because of the claim that it increases sexual potency, but actually it does the opposite. It has been touted for relief of fatigue, cure for heart disease and leg pains, and many other things. Vitamin E can cause headache, nausea, blurring of vision, chapped lips, muscle weakness, and bleeding as well as low blood sugar. Dr. R. J. Shephard and associates of the Department of Environmental Health, School of Hygiene, University of Toronto, tested vitamin E on swimmers, giving them 1200 international units a day for 85 days and using paired controls—half using vitamin E and half placebos. The fact that there was no difference in the groups showed that vitamin E does not cause increased energy.

Every major medical study has shown no vitamin E deficiency state in humans, nor any benefit derived from taking it. In another double-blind study made in 1974, eight healthy young male volunteers were fed 800 international units of vitamin E daily. Severe fatigue and weakness caused three to drop out after three weeks. These were three of those who took the vitamin E. Those on placebos felt well. Between 1953 and 1961 there was a study made in Elgin State Hospital in Illinois under the auspices of the Food and Nutrition Board of the National Research Council. After six years of diets very low in vitamin E there was no change in the physical or mental status of the subjects studied. Other studies at Mount Sinai Hospital in New York, the University of Manchester in England, Duke University School of Medicine in North Carolina, and many others confirmed that vitamin E did not effect any benefit to angina patients or those having any other form of heart disease.*

All of the vitamins, in excess, can disturb blood values of sugar, uric acid, and enzymes. With nothing to gain and so much to lose, do you think that this fad is rational?

In Appendix D, you will find an example of calorie estimation as a scientist would do it. I have also included my "Thirteen Day Diet" in Appendix C because it has proved so successful and popular over the years. Most people lose six to ten pounds in the thirteen days.

I wish all you weight-losers would ask your physicians for a pamphlet called "Are You Really Serious about Losing Weight," published by Pennwalt and written by Dr. Jean Mayer, professor of nutrition at the Harvard University's School of Public Health. Copies can be obtained through your family physician. It shows that popular diets which make unreasonable promises to people do not emphasize the all-important fact that you have to reduce the food you take in and increase the energy you put out. This means that you have to revise your eating habits through retraining.

The pamphlet explodes many myths about eating and weight. It starts with a quiz to see how much you know about eating. For example, is it true or false that "Fat should be eliminated in a reducing diet"? Answer: "False. Some fat is necessary for its nutrient value as well as for its satiety value in staving off hunger." Another: "Exercise increases the appetite." Answer: "False. Moderate exercise, done regularly, is a regulator of body weight. It does not increase the appetite in the overweight person. Activity is a good way to use up calories and keep the body physically fit. In many obese persons, the beginning of obesity can be traced to decreased activity." And another: "Overweight people are generally happy, healthy people." Answer: "False. In actual fact, overweight people are much more content after they have lost their excess fat. They become unhappy if they regain the weight they lost. Insurance figures have proven that overweight persons have a shorter life expectancy and are more susceptible to cardiovascular and degenerative diseases." One more: "Alcohol, even though not a protein, fat, or carbohydrate, furnishes calories to the body." Answer: "True. Alcohol has no nutritive value. Therefore, alcohol is used by the body only as a source of calories (energy). An equivalent number of food calories become surplus, however, and are stored as fat. Few people realize that a large whiskey or gin, or a pint of beer, is the caloric equivalent of two eggs, or one glass of milk, or a slice of bread and butter, or an average portion of potatoes."

---

*Vitamin E: Miracle or Myth?. *Nutrition Review* Suppl: 35, 32 (July 1974): 35.

The pamphlet explains why your weight drops irregularly, even though you are dieting steadily; discusses water retention; why "crash" diets are inadvisable; the importance of rest as well as exercise; how it takes a month to retrain the appetite so that you are satisfied with less food; the calorie value of foods; calories burned during various activities; and much more.

Many low-calorie foods can be substituted for high-calorie ones. They taste just as good and you don't even feel that you are dieting, yet your intake is reduced from 4000 to 2000 calories per day. This is the basis of long-term success in dieting.

Do You Know About Triglycerides?

Triglycerides come mainly from two sources: the *rich carbohydrates*—such as chocolate, ice cream, sweets of all kinds, and refined sugars; and from *saturated animal fats*—such as marbled beef, pork, chicken skin, and artificial dairy creamers. The importance of triglycerides is still being debated; they may play a role, although a lesser one, in the causation of coronary artery disease. (It is necessary to fast some fourteen hours before the test is taken to establish significant levels.) A recent study compared one hundred patients with coronary artery disease, proved by X rays of the arteries, with one hundred normals, proved in the same way. The level of triglycerides was insignificant except when the cholesterol count was also elevated. So triglyceride elevation by itself is not nearly as important as other coronary risk factors, and may even be unimportant except when accompanied by high cholesterol level. Additionally, it should be noted that there is no critical level of either one. However, it is generally agreed that exercise has a favorable and consistent effect on lowering both fasting triglyceride levels and the rise which occurs after eating.

Will Your "Type A" Personality Kill You?

Drs. Meyer Friedman and R. H. Rosenman (both from Harold Brunn Institute, Mount Zion Hospital and Medical Center, San Francisco, California) have written a book called *Type A Behavior and Your Heart*. They describe the person who is always pressured by a sense of time, always under tension to do more things than he has time for, who is aggressive, competitive, and impatient. They call this the "hurry sickness":

> It is the Type A man's ceaseless striving, his everlasting struggle with time, that we believe so very frequently leads to his early demise from coronary heart disease. . . . Perhaps the prime index of the presence of aggression or hostility in almost all Type A men

is the tendency always to compete with or to challenge other people, whether the activity consists of a sporting contest, a game of cards, or a simple discussion.

They believe that such men have hormonal abnormalities that raise their blood cholesterols (here we go again), which, with increased clotting of the blood, leads to damaged blood vessels and premature heart attacks. They also state that strenuous exercise past the age of thirty-five is dangerous: "First on our blacklist is jogging." They advise a search for "aloneness," long periods of solitude, subduing the desire for material things and cultivating spiritual virtues.

If you can't succeed in altering your behavior pattern, you aren't being protected against heart disease, no matter how little cholesterol you now eat, how little cigarette smoke you inhale, or how many miles you run each day.

Actually, they do advise their coronary patients to walk every day. In 1976, in a more recent report, they followed over three thousand middle-aged men for more than eight years. Coronary artery disease was related to cholesterol, behavior pattern, smoking, blood pressure, and age. The authors felt that Type A behavior was a strong factor in all age groups, but they admitted that there were many unknown factors yet to be discovered before accurate predictions could be made.

I think it would be foolish to deny that individuals exist whose personalities contribute to their development of disease, but it should be pointed out that this hypothesis is not proved, and it is a pretty dismal prospect to believe that there is nothing one can do to avert a heart attack if you can't change your personality. Nor have the authors shown that those who have purportedly changed have been able to avert heart disease. As to their attitude toward exercise, this whole book offers refutation. Here is some more evidence from two of our leading exercise physiologists who were also interested in psychosocial factors.

Exercise Is an Antidote to Compulsive Drive

John P. Naughton and Herman K. Hellerstein have studied the influence of psychosocial factors on coronary risk in relation to exercise. These factors are the Type A personality, the self-esteem in which the individual holds himself, and his social position. The factors were then related to a program of physical fitness. There are ways of determining who is a Type A individual and of estimating his personality; that is, does he present himself in a favorable or unfavorable manner? The personality test determines such things as sexual activity, drive, income level, number of children, success, and the like. The study showed that the low-esteem individual of *low excitability* was a higher coronary risk. It was concluded that the influence of the Type A personality could not be proved, but if the person had risk factors making him subject to heart attack, *these could be lessened by exercise.*

Are There Precursors of Premature Disease and Death?

The psychological, social, and behavioral factors associated with the risk of coronary disease have been thoroughly reviewed. Increased coronary disease is twice as high among white-collar workers as farmers. Certain occupations as well as degree of physical activity are contributory factors. For example, fire fighters, despite low incidence of coronary-risk factors (since they were a selected group), exhibit a very high percent of abnormal exercise tests, suggesting that their heart disease is job-related.

Dr. C. B. Thomas (of the Department of Medicine, John Hopkins University School of Medicine, Baltimore, Maryland) has found evidence that psychological traits in youth which may precede premature disease and even death from heart disease, high blood pressure, mental disease, and cancer can be determined. In the coronary-prone medical student, followed and diligently observed over thirty years, Dr. Thomas found such traits as unusual nervous tension, being tired on awakening, insomnia, becoming angry under stress, and so on. There were different factors involved in other premature diseases. The point is that there may well be some kind of relation between psychological traits and the circumstances under which certain individuals become ill while others remain well. Here, again, the tension-relieving ability of exercise could modify personality characteristics and stress.

Nonmarried people have more heart attacks than married ones. Churchgoers suffer fewer attacks than those who stay away from places of worship. Why? Nobody knows for sure.

It has been found that men who have severe problems with their families or their co-workers suffered 2.5 times the rate of angina as those who had no problems in these areas. Some investigators have called this "psychosocial discord." In a study of Swedish twins, financial worries preceded by several years the onset of heart pain, but for reasons that are not understood, a heart attack was not definitely associated with these factors. We have much to learn in these areas, and I do not believe that at this stage of our knowledge it is possible to predict what kind of diseases will afflict unhappy people.

It is often difficult to distinguish between stress and achievement as illustrated by H. C. Lehman's 1943 study of chess players and other professionals. Champion chess requires intense effort and great physical stamina. It was found that the average life span of thirty-two outstanding players was sixty years. Morphy, Capablanca, and Alekhine died of strokes between forty-five and fifty-five years of age. None of them engaged in any real physical activity. Chess players with other interests have lived longer than those whose only interest was chess, and the lesser chess players have lived ten years longer than the world champions.

Lehman also studied twenty-four other occupations. Of 248 members of presidents' cabinets, the average age at death was seventy-one; for 543 British authors, it was sixty-four. Corporate executives have a favorable mortality rate over the general average of their contemporaries, often by as much as 30 percent. This probably reflects the physical and emotional fitness of executives for coping with stressful situations, their work satisfactions, and recognition of accomplishment. Studies show that men of high professional and business achievement—"strivers"—have a comparatively low mortality rate.

A device called a quiz electrocardiogram is being used to test for the effect of emotional stress on the heart. Heart rate and blood pressure go up while the subject is attempting to answer harder and harder questions. Executives with heart pain showed much more rise in pulse and blood pressure than those who had no angina.

John M. Rhoads of the Department of Psychiatry, Duke University Medical Center has drawn attention to the "overwork syndrome." In 1894 the average workweek lasted 58 hours; now it is about 40 hours, but people in average jobs, because of stress, guilt feelings, the inability to relax or depression, will drive themselves as though they were working in a sweatshop. He cites cases of people who develop fatigue, sleep disturbances, irritability, inability to concentrate, memory losses, confusional episodes, and disturbances in their gastrointestinal and cardiovascular systems simulating disease. Treatment involves an evaluation of the person's attitude toward work. Here again an activity oriented toward physical fitness can contribute immensely to a restoration of the balance of work-rest-recreation.

George M. Hass (professor in the Department of Pathology, Rush Presbyterian, St. Luke's Medical Center, Chicago) has determined that when only one or two coronary-risk factors are present, they are relatively harmless. It is the *combination of risk factors* which is important.

People who become unduly alarmed over some minor abnormality remind me of a medical-school classmate of mine. Whenever he read the description of a disease, he was sure he had it and would run to the professor in great agitation. One day the professor, a bit irritated by these repeated visits, was heard to say, "You know, Jack, some day you are going to die of a misprint!"

So You Still Smoke!

Cigarette smoking is firmly established as an important determinant of coronary mortality, which is certainly related to the amount smoked (Americans smoked 603 *billion* cigarettes in 1975; 565 billion in 1972), but ten years went by before it was realized that mortality rates were dropping as a result of the American Heart Association's condemnation of smoking. Middle-aged people were kicking the habit, but many young people still became addicted. Importantly, smoking itself does not usually cause heart pain, and I have found, particularly in women patients, that an exercise test is needed to diagnose coronary disease in those who have smoked more than one pack a day for over twenty years. There is at least one hopeful fact: If you stop smoking before you're sixty-five, you cut the risk of coronary disease by half. It is never too late to start exercising or to stop smoking. According to Alton Ochsner (of the Ochsner Clinic, New Orleans; recipient of the 1976 Edward Henderson Gold Medal award of the American Geriatrics Society), the three most important factors that accelerate aging are tobacco, particularly cigarettes; lack of exercise; and excess weight. The latest figures indicate that the risks for pipe and cigar smokers are no less than those for cigarette smokers.

A 1975 Health, Education and Welfare survey of smoking showed that fifteen years of warnings had convinced 80 percent of smokers that what they were doing was harmful, yet 57 percent were still smoking. Ninety percent of smokers want to stop, but most of these have not been able to quit. Dr. John Farquhar heads a research program at Stanford University Medical Center. He, as well as other investigators from the American Cancer Society, have found that the first fault is with the physician, who does not make emphatic enough statements against smoking or point out during the physical exam the symptoms associated with smoking, such as fatigue, breathlessness, and palpitation. In my office, we perform a breathing test and can show the patient on a graph his lessening ability to move air in and out.

As to the programs that are designed to help the patient stop smoking, most investigators feel that the help comes from the mutual aid people give to one another when they meet to solve a common problem—like Alcoholics Anonymous. The success rate varies between 10 and 40 percent. Where such programs fail, the person often becomes so discouraged that he never tries to quit again. When I have convinced someone by a chest X-ray, a breathing test, or an exercise electrocardiogram that smoking is already leading him to bronchitis, emphysema, heart disease, and cancer, and he throws his cigarette package in my waste basket, he usually quits for good. But when he is going to start quitting tomorrow, or to "cut down," I know I have failed. Dr. Donald T. Frederickson, who is an associate professor of public health at New York University School of Medicine, puts it bluntly: "Lots of people don't need clinics but a boot in the rear end."

Some Good News

It has been substantiated that coffee and alcohol do not cause coronary artery disease. Dr. K. Yano and associates have shown in the Honolulu Heart Study that alcohol in small amounts, up to 2 ounces per day, particularly beer, seems to actually lower the risk of heart attack. Large amounts of alcohol, however, can damage the heart. Similarly, coffee in the absence of cigarettes also constitutes no risk. Blood uric acid is definitely an important factor, but high uric acid is one of the most easily controlled risk factors. We can use one medicine to cause the kidneys to get rid of uric acid, or we can use another to reduce the amount made in the body, and we can usually allow you to eat a normal diet.

Does Physical Fitness Combat Coronary Risk Factors?

We understand many of the factors producing coronary heart disease very well, and we have many effective weapons for its treatment. But most of all, we want to prevent it, and if we can't do that, then we at least want to detect it before there is an attack. This is certainly possible now for the majority—if patients cooperate and if doctors use the available methods for detection.

A recent study of three thousand men, average age forty-five, looked at the known coronary-risk factors and then correlated the men's degree of physical fitness. The fit had lower blood pressures; slower heart rates; lower cholesterol, triglycerides, and sugars; leaner body weight; greater breathing capacity and endurance—that is, the more fit, the lower the factors producing sudden death and heart attack.

As to what our master has mentioned regarding weakness after exercise, the cause of this is its omission. If he resumes it gradually, little by little, he will find following it the strength and the vitality that should be found after all exercise that is carried out properly.

Maimonides, 1198

Chapter 8.
Rehabilitation of the Heart Attack Patient

A heart attack is a tremendous blow to a person's self-esteem, economic status and earning capacity, and physical capability. It is normal to become depressed under these circumstances. To suffer the terrors of a coronary-care unit, to be invaded through almost every orifice, to tolerate the violation of privacy and modesty, and to endure pain and the fear of death induces despair and fear in anyone.

The physician is aware of all this, and from the earliest moment of treatment, seeks to ameliorate these traumas to the body and spirit. Most patients are nevertheless left with great uncertainties about how to rehabilitate themselves and are troubled by many misconceptions, which they often keep to themselves, such as the fear that sexual intercourse can cause another heart attack. They believe they may never be able to undergo even mild exertion. Nothing could be more inaccurate or interfere more with recovery.

Exercise Builds Confidence

A carefully planned exercise program does far more than promote physical fitness. Physiologist Lange Anderson believes the benefit of exercise is more psychological than physiological, and Dr. S. M. Fox has emphasized its tranquillizing quality. Certainly it helps in combating depression, promoting confidence, and eliminating fear. When a post-coronary patient can walk a fifteen-minute mile (three miles in forty-five minutes), feel vigorous and exhilarated afterward, get on the treadmill and turn in a superior performance, he has been rehabilitated. Many patients say, "Thank God for my heart attack," meaning that they have learned a better way of life both physically and philosophically.

Over and over again, I have seen patients who had two or three heart attacks in the space of a few years begin an exercise program, persist with it, grow vigorous, and remain symptom-free for many years. And often the only coronary-risk factor that was changed was lack of exercise.

Recovery Period Requires Special Vigilance

The immediate postcoronary period is a particularly vulnerable time during which careful supervision must be made of any activity. Studies have shown that patients having skip beats during this period may have more serious rhythm disturbances, and that sudden death can occur in such patients.

This period may last up to six months after heart attack and should be managed with appropriate medications. Certainly no patient should be allowed strenuous activity during this time without careful testing, preferably monitoring during exercise.

Rehabilitation Programs

Many hospitals, teaching institutions, YMCAs, and physical educators now offer rehabilitation programs. These programs are necessary to instruct and support the patient during the period when he is most dependent. However, the average physician can accomplish the objective of making the patient strong and independent through a progressive walking program. It is no different, basically, from the regimen offered to the normal but sedentary person who is out of condition and seeking physical fitness. The individual sets his own pace, taking care not to overtax the recovering heart muscle, but is made to walk progressively faster as time passes.

The criteria for entrance into an exercise program have been well established. At the outset, certain patients with heart disease must be excluded. But surprisingly, in most of the subjects tested, there were few who could not participate in a program of exercise conditioning. By the time a patient is recovered enough to walk around his house (two to four weeks after hospitalization), he is ready to take a slow ten-minute walk. Each day or so he adds a minute, attempting to build up the time to an hour without regard to distance. Later, when he walks for an hour without fatigue or other symptoms, he measures the distance in his car and slowly attempts to walk three miles in one hour. When he can do this, he is ready for an exercise test. If he has recovered enough, I then have him gradually reduce the time until he is covering the three miles in forty-five minutes—that is, a fifteen-minute mile.

Experience with this program for over two decades has convinced me that a patient can maintain a high degree of physical fitness at this level. If he plays golf, he can omit his walks on this day, thus averaging only three to four walking days a week.

L. S. is a lawyer from Chicago, the brother of another good friend and patient. He came to me in despair in 1964, when he was fifty-nine years old. He had been hospitalized for four heart attacks—in '53, '60, '63, and '64. He could not walk a block without pain and shortness of breath. In six months of progressive walking, he was able to cover three miles in the morning and two miles in the afternoon at a pace of fifteen minutes per mile. He has now done this almost daily for twelve years—he is now seventy-one—feels fine, and passes a standard exercise test with ease. No other risk factor has been corrected. Neither he nor his wife, who walks with him for her coronary disease, believes this result is coincidence.

Take Your Nitro to *Prevent* Pain

Some patients experience angina either midway or toward the end of exercise. They are taught to anticipate and prevent this by taking nitroglycerin before exercising, since experience has shown this to occur. This opens up the vessels immediately rather than waiting for the effect of exercise, and avoids the chest pressure and the insufficient coronary flow occasioned by the change from rest to exercise before the heart has a chance to adapt. If they do not use nitroglycerin, they can often "walk through" this mild pain period, as Dr. Albert Kattus has shown in his studies at UCLA, but it's better to prevent pain and spare the heart this additional strain.

Nearly all patients are resistant to taking nitroglycerin and would rather bear the mild discomfort or sensation of an angina attack. They may say, "It doesn't last long enough," or "It doesn't really hurt." But the cardiologist knows the benefits of nitro in reducing the requirements of the heart for oxygen and in promoting better coronary flow. Here are the instructions I give my patients in order to break down this resistance and teach them how to use nitroglycerin most effectively.

How to Use Nitroglycerin

Nitroglycerin for medical use is one of the greatest discoveries for patients with chest pain due to angina pectoris or coronary artery disease. This is the kind of pain or pressure or uncomfortable sensation in the chest, arms, shoulder, neck, or jaw brought on by exertion, emotion, excitement, eating, and the like. The pain is the result of an inadequate blood flow to the heart, which is relieved by placing nitro (1/150 of a grain) under the tongue. The nitro has the effect of dilating the heart arteries and allowing more blood flow.

Its action is quick—thirty to forty seconds—and produces a tingling sensation under the tongue, a feeling of flushing or throbbing, and sometimes a transient headache. Such side effects show that the tablets are working and are potent; the absence of such side effects usually means that the tablets are too old and have lost their kick. Nitro ages fast because it volatilizes—evaporates—and must be kept by itself in a tightly stopped container. A new supply should be obtained—nitro is inexpensive—when the tablets cannot be easily crushed between the fingers.

Nitro can be used repeatedly in almost any amount for the relief of pain. When chest pain is relieved promptly, you know that you are safe. When it persists after using two or three fresh tablets, the doctor should be notified. *Do not use nitro except for chest or arm pressure or pain. If you feel faint, for example, it could make you worse.*

Nitro should also be used freely to prevent chest discomfort provoked by activities known by experience to have this effect. This prophylactic use is highly protective.

Nitroglycerin is not really an explosive, but it does evaporate quickly and a fresh supply is necessary. Long-acting drugs having the same action are also in common use, and new ones are rapidly being developed, but none is so quick and effective as nitroglycerin.

J. A., one of my tennis partners, had an operation for heart trouble; in fact, he had the old Vineberg operation of internal mammary artery implantation ten years ago, before the bypass operation of modern times was adopted. Still a young man, he plays tennis vigorously almost every day. He completes a full treadmill exercise test without any abnormality or angina, but when he begins to play, he often experiences some pressure. He may also feel it when he serves hard during an exciting game. Now he has grown accustomed to taking nitroglycerin before he starts to play and to repeat this before his turn to serve, and he avoids any onslaught of angina. When testing him on the court, we could find no abnormality. He gave up golf because he felt it was not a good enough exercise, and he attributes his present good health to playing tennis.

Consult Your Doctor at Least Once a Year

Serious abnormalities can occur even in apparently normal people *without their knowledge*. There are those with advanced disease who are subject to dangerous arrhythmias, not to mention the untold number of people with undiagnosed diabetes, coronary artery disease, and hypertension. Exercise, high altitudes, and even everyday activities, such as automobile driving, can cause silent arrhythmias.

T. F., a friend who came to play tennis, mentioned that he had an uncomfortable pressure in his chest. I advised him not to play until he saw his doctor. He informed me that he had not seen a doctor in ten years. On examination, he was found to have severe high blood pressure, and an exercise electrocardiogram showed it to be of the type that threatened acute heart attack or sudden death. Yet he had been playing for months with no indication of disease.

The rehabilitation program which I have recommended for years to those who have had heart attacks is outlined below:

Instructions for Progressive Exercise

> *Method*
> Begin by walking steadily at your own pace on level ground. Later you may swim, bicycle, use a treadmill at a ten-degree incline, and, in selected instances, run or engage in more strenuous sports.
>
> *Requirements*
> 1. At first *walk on level ground*.
> 2. Exercise only on an empty stomach—at least two hours after a meal.
> 3. Avoid inclement weather; do not get chilled or overheated. Wear comfortable shoes and loose clothing.
> 4. Patients with angina should always take nitroglycerin before starting out and at any point where experience shows chest pressure may begin.
> 5. Count your resting heart rate and the rate just at the end of exercise. Note any irregularity; bring these reports when you come in for your checkup.
> 6. Walk for a specific time. Distances come later. Start at any comfortable period; for example, ten minutes at your own pace. Avoid fatigue, breathlessness, pain, or weakness. Each day or so, at your discretion, increase by one minute until an hour's walk is achieved. Remember what you have learned

about Dash Training and alternate your pace—walk fast and slow—at 30 second to two-minute intervals, and swing your arms to increase the exercise value.

7. Next, measure the distance in your car. Then try to walk three miles in one hour (twenty minutes per mile). If it takes you more than an hour to cover the distance, gradually reduce the time.

8. Come in for an exercise test on the treadmill at this point. The doctor will determine your training heart rate and your capability of advancing.

9. If the test is satisfactory, begin to shave minutes off the hour until you can walk the three miles in forty-five minutes *easily*. Two-minute run-walk sequences can be started here.

10. For those who wish to do strenuous sports involving running and sudden effort, testing in advance is required. This will include going from rest to four miles per hour. For sudden-effort sports like tennis, you may be required to wear a monitor during actual play.

11. To maintain fitness, you must continue the degree of exercise achieved at your training heart rate for at least thirty minutes three times a week.

S. S. is a man of many achievements. He suffered a heart attack at the age of forty-eight. He was a fine golfer, but at the age of fifty-five, because of the development of angina, he turned to tennis, hoping to strengthen his heart and "work out" the angina. Within a year, effort no longer caused pain in his chest and he could pass an exercise test. But, because of business pressures, he failed to exercise consistently. During an annual physical exam, he did poorly on his exercise test and was told of his deterioration. This spurred him to renewed efforts. He became lean and trim, and played tennis either with his pro or his friends several times a week. When he was reexamined only six months later, he went through an advanced exercise test with no evidence of disease; and the systolic time intervals (see chapter 12, "More About Exercise Testing") indicated a vigorously contracting heart with no evidence of impaired flow. Moreover, in a tennis test during singles, he had an excellent score (he was now sixty-six). This example illustrates the improvement that can be attained by a persistent program, as well as the decline that ensues when exercise is neglected.

There are Many Ways to Achieve Fitness

Walking is tedious for some people, or they may find the thirty to forty-five minutes—two hours after a meal—difficult to arrange. Some of these people elect to use home treadmills or other devices. I have found that the roller type home treadmills are inexpensive and practical. They can be set at a ten-degree grade and have speed indicators that go up at least four miles per hour. I insist on the level walking program first, but will then allow those who perform well during the exercise test to go on to the home treadmill. At this point they can progressively increase the time and speed to four miles per hour for twenty minutes and because of the increased workload maintain the same degree of physical fitness as by the thirty-minute, two-mile walk at the training heart rate. The treadmill can be set in front of the television set to relieve boredom.

Jogging Is Different from Running

For those who want to go beyond the two-mile walk, an advanced exercise test is required. They must be able to do at least five miles per hour on the treadmill without strain. Jogging has become popular, but it doesn't mean the same thing to everyone. To some, it's a slow run; to others, it means alternate walking and running; and still others refer to a stiff-legged, jarring trot. This punishing gait has been shown by orthopedists to injure hip and knee joints and by opthalmologists to cause retinal detachment. Gynecologists think it causes the uterus to drop. Orthopedists recognize that there is a great deal of difference between the jarring trot and the long, loping gait of running. Orthopedic complications in the locomotive system have been reported in 50 percent of participants in jogging programs. A cause of death in jogging programs is underlying coronary-artery disease in patients who were unsupervised, unconditioned and uneducated in the proper way to jog, as pointed out by Dr. N. Kuller.

Too Much Leg Fatigue from Bicycle Devices

There are other methods of exercise such as using stationary bicycles with adjustable pedal resistance, mechanical joggers, and the like. While these are useful, Americans are not like Scandinavians, who are accustomed to doing vigorous leg exercises from childhood on. My patients usually get leg fatigue before the heart is sufficiently stressed (before they reach their target heart rates) and do not achieve equal levels of physical fitness attained by other methods.

Isometrics Are Not the Way

Isometric exercise can be deleterious. President Eisenhower is said to have sustained his heart attack while attempting to open a stuck window, an act which involves isometriclike activity. Isometric (muscle tension without motion) as opposed to kinetic (muscle tension with motion) exercise raises blood pressure and intracardiac pressures, sometimes to dangerous levels with little or no change in the amount of blood pumped with each stroke. You can prove this by squeezing your fist tightly. More over, endurance is not increased and at higher work loads the heart is working with very little oxygen. There have been reports of sudden death during waterskiing, probably because this sport is an intense form of isometrics. The heart attack patient should not try to lift heavy weights or push or strain heavily, especially during bowel movements. Action games and sports are more desirable if the precautions necessary for participating in sudden-effort sports are taken, because here the increase in heart rate and blood per stroke (cardiac output) is large.

When Can the Heart Attack Patient Play Running Sports?

The use of sports training in the rehabilitation of the cardiac patient is not new. Dr. Victor Gottheiner, mentioned earlier, has been using it on several thousand Israeli patients since 1955. He has preferred brisk walking, running, cycling, swimming, rowing, and volley ball. No deaths occurred during supervised training. The mortality rate for the exercise group over a five-year period was 3.6 percent as compared to a 12 percent mortality in physically inactive post-heart attack patients.

Before permitting a heart attack patient to play running sports, I first require him to undertake a graduated physical-fitness program and achieve satisfactory performance at the four-mile-per-hour level of walking. Then he must not only pass an advanced exercise test at the five-mile-per-hour level requiring running, but, in addition, he must be able to go from rest to four miles per hour for at least thirty seconds without developing symptoms or manifesting signs of heart weakness. In doubtful cases, he is monitored during the sports activity by a portable device.

Obviously there are patients who develop chest pains, shortness of breath, severe fatigue, faintness, drop in blood pressure, arrhythmias, and electrocardiographic and systolic time-interval abnormalities who cannot be permitted strenuous activities. Surprisingly, however, the majority who will follow a disciplined training program are able to play safely and with enjoyment. Dr. Terrence Kavanaugh, medical director of the Toronto Cardiac Rehabilitation Center, trained eight middle-aged heart attack patients for the 1974 Boston Marathon. Seven of the eight completed the entire race, running at about 5.4 miles per hour, in remarkably good condition. Although this type of exercise is not recommended for most victims of heart attack, it demonstrates what can be achieved. While the times and distances recommended for the walking rehabilitation program have evolved from my own experience, they are in surprising agreement with other studies.

Most Seriously Damaged Patients Can be Rehabilitated

Rehabilitation programs are not always 100 percent successful. A survey of 1,350 patients by Dr. John Naughton, dean, State University of New York at Buffalo School of Medicine, and associates revealed twenty deaths, but *none* occurred during exercise. (Most occurred at night.) One cannot deal with heart-injured patients without expecting, in the natural history of the disease, that some will have arrhythmias, recurrent heart attacks, heart failures, and so forth. Some will require bypass surgery because their medical programs will not rehabilitate them. In general, however, even with advanced disease, studies have shown that 80 percent can be rehabilitated through a training program.

The first scientific study of regular exercise for the coronary patient was reported in the United States by Dr. Herman Hellerstein in 1963, although many years previously, Dr. Paul D. White had advocated exercise to the point of breathlessness.

The most recent review of the rehabilitation of the heart attack patient has come from Israel. Dr. Jan J. Kellerman (Chaim Sheba Medical School, Tel Hashomer Medical School, University of Israel) followed up on patients with and without angina for twelve years after a heart attack. Of those who did not undergo a program of exercise, *29 percent* died of recurrent heart attack. Of those who undertook a short training program of thirty to seventy months, *33 percent* died. But of those who maintained a continuous program, *only 9 percent died*. Perhaps such studies are not conclusive, but they afford positive evidence that a persistent exercise program is beneficial for the heart attack patient. Certainly exercise is not *increasing* the mortality rate. Physiologically and psychologically, there seems to be no controversy about the salutary results; moreover, it seems well established that the same beneficial effects of exercise achieved by the normal person can be duplicated in the heart attack patient.

Who Wants to Wait a Hundred Years?

While it is admitted that more evidence is needed to convince everyone that heart patients who exercise live longer or have fewer coronary episodes, all are agreed that the quality of their lives is greatly enriched.

Authorities speculate that it may take a hundred years or more of intensive research to find conclusive answers. I for one do not want to wait that long. I made this decision over twenty years ago and am now more convinced than ever. Even among patients who exercised and still required bypass surgery, the accessory vessels and the increased size of the vessels below the obstruction made the surgery easier and more successful.

*To fear love is to fear life, and those who fear life are
already three parts dead.*

Bertrand Russell, 1929

Chapter 9.
Sex and Your Heart

Discussions of sexual activity as it relates to the heart have been sparse in
medical literature. The subject is often passed off with a joke when a
convalescent patient finally gets up his courage to ask the doctor if intercourse is now permissible. The stock answer is, "Yes, but just with your
wife; I don't want you to get too excited." Of late, however, the subject is
more prominent in medical publications. Patients are often afraid that the
effort of sex is dangerous and that orgasm can kill. Be happy! That isn't
true.

Sex Is Not Work

Physiological studies have been made during intercourse. In one study
on middle-aged men, reported by Michael Sketch and David Turner (of the
Cardiac Laboratory, Omaha), the average peak heart rate was 117 and was
maintained for thirty seconds. This was only 70 percent of their capabilities. It was concluded that the heart rate and the degree of work involved is less than half the individual's capacity—about equal to climbing a
flight of stairs. This was true of the recovered heart attack patient as well as
the normal man. Questionnaires have also revealed that sex is pursued by
the average male about twice a week.

It has been shown that males and females "turn on" at about the same
time—three to fifteen seconds, as determined by erection or lubrication
time. Maximum heart rate may not be reached for sixteen minutes, but 74
percent of males reach their maximum rates at orgasm in under ten
minutes. For thirty seconds, they are burning six calories per minute—

about the same as doubles tennis or walking three miles per hour—and within two minutes they are down to burning 4.5 calories. Orgasm itself lasts only about ten seconds! Sex, therefore, must be classed as a mild exercise of short duration.

Dash Training Is Good for Sex

Studies have been made of patients who underwent Dash Training after heart attack with respect to their peak heart rates and oxygen consumption during sexual intercourse. According to Dr. Richard Stein, the exercise-trained group showed improved sexual function in terms of lower heart rates and improved oxygen consumption, as compared to similar patients who did not exercise.

Some patients have asked me if sex could substitute as a training program! Unfortunately for the average person, the activity is all too brief to qualify.

Is Intercourse Hazardous to the Cardiac Patient?

A recent report by Dr. R. H. Rosenman examined only those heart attack patients who required resuscitation for recovery. Even here it was found that the ability to perform sexually was unimpaired. Electrocardiographic changes recorded during coitus are no different from those during ordinary activities. A person who can pass a standard exercise test has worked much harder during the test than he does during intercourse. Drs. John Naughton's and Herman Hellerstein's studies have shown that 80 percent of coronary disease patients—even those with advanced disease—can be rehabilitated through a training program. For the patient with angina, nitroglycerin should be taken prophylactically—and some say it heightens the orgasmic thrill.

Death during sex does occur, but only rarely. Talk about it has engendered more fear in the female partner than in the male cardiac patient. Often she is asked to play the aggressive role and, as a result, sexual activity may be avoided. Monitoring by an electrocardiogram during intercourse can be used if such fears are intense, but an exercise test, particularly the sudden-effort type, affords ample protection. Heart attack among females during intercourse is particularly rare.

Fear Reduces Desire

A study of patients of both sexes who had recovered from a heart attack revealed that the average monthly frequency of sexual intercourse was 5.2 before the attack. Eleven months after the episode, the monthly frequency averaged only 2.7, despite resumption of normal life in all other respects. Exercise tests showed no correlation between work capacity and the frequency of intercourse. A questionnaire that tried to find the reasons for the reduction of sexual activity came up with these answers: diminished desire, depression, anxiety, wife's decision, fear of recurrence or death, fatigue, angina, and impotence. However, impotence was the reason given by only one respondent. The main reason for the drop in frequency was not physical but psychological—fear! The fear was of sudden death or recurrence, particularly at orgasm. Frank discussion in most instances was able to overcome this fear so that there was a return to normal frequency.

When death during sex does occur, there is usually a pattern: The male is married, but is with a "nonspouse" in strange surroundings, after a big meal and intoxicating amounts of alcohol.

Drs. A. M. Master and H. L. Jaffe studied the setting preceding heart attack and demonstrated that most occurred at rest or sleep, and only 8 percent occurred during moderate activity, including intercourse. The number that occurred during unusual exertion was 2 percent.

Doctors themselves have contributed to this unfounded fear. A questionnaire on heart disease and sex showed the following recommendations by physicians to patients after heart attack: limited sex—83 percent; abstinence for two to twelve weeks—50 percent; unlimited sex—13 percent. Seventy percent of the doctors believed there was a real hazard, and only 31 percent would discuss the subject. It is time for all doctors to deal with this fear realistically and eradicate it from their patients. In questioning my own patients, I find that the realization that they have passed an exacting exercise test is very reassuring. Many of them who have been trained to count their heart rates after exertion report that their rates after intercourse are not as high as after activities such as tennis, and they have no fear at all. They understand what is meant by the training heart rate and appreciate that at the level after intercourse, they are well below their maximum capacity. They know also that their heart rhythms show no irregularities. Confidence comes from knowledge and observation, not from an offhand pat on the back.

Sex for the Elderly

Many elderly people have retarded ejaculation so that coitus may be prolonged. Some women prefer older men because erection is sustained and they can have multiple orgasms. Even such men need not fear excessive cardiovascular strain unless they are trying to impress their partners with their sexual vigor and force themselves into "explosive orgasms."

On the other hand, there are some misinformed people who think sexual activity should be curtailed or reduced after the age of sixty-five. Surveys show that at age sixty-eight, 70 percent of men are still sexually active, and at age seventy-eight at least 25 percent are active. Sexual interest plays a significant role in a person's life-style and contributes greatly to the satisfactions of older persons.

Nearly all who have studied sexual activity in the aging male or female find a high percentage of interest and capacity in people up to one hundred years or more. The physical capacity may decline somewhat but is still present. And it does appear true that those who remain sexually active are most apt to continue their interest and ability. Since opportunity and morality also figure in the total picture, it is more common to find activity in the male than in the female. There are more sexually active unmarried males than females for these reasons.

One of my patients with a heart murmur plays tennis every day for at least thirty minutes. He is unmarried but always has a young girl friend in tow. He is now eighty-two years old and is always coming in for me to test him because he has intercourse three to four times a week and is worried that he may strain his heart. I put a Holter (electrocardiographic monitor) on him during coitus. He took sixteen minutes to reach orgasm at a maximal heart rate of 128, without any evidence of abnormality. At doubles tennis, his heart rate goes to 136, and he occasionally has to take nitroglycerin for mild angina. But he says he never has angina during intercourse.

Does Sex Sap Your Energy?

A question that is often asked is, What effect does sexual intercourse have on subsequent athletic performance? Will it improve performance, as some have claimed, because it relieves tension? Or will it sap your energy? There seem to be no precise studies on this subject, but it has been reported that most athletes state that it does relieve their anxieties. Certainly there is no evidence that energy is depleted even in those who masturbate before athletic competition.

G. B. was a nineteen-year-old miler who was a star on the track team. He found that he was much less tense if he had sex with his girl friend before competition, but he worried that he would not be able to run as well. I put a heart monitor on him. During intercourse, his peak rate was 96 (resting, 42). At the end of the race, his rate was 172, and on this occasion he won the race! I have not heard from him since.

There is a disorder of the breast marked with strong and peculiar symptoms, considerable for the kind of danger belonging to it, and not extremely rare, which deserves to be mentioned more at length. The seat of it, and sense of strangling, and anxiety with which it is attended, may make it not improperly be called angina pectoris.

William Heberden, 1818

Chapter 10.
Bypass Heart Surgery

The popularity of bypass surgery for life-threatening coronary disease is burgeoning. Some medical centers perform a great number of such operations a day. The reason for considering the subject here is that some people are beginning to think that surgery replaces a medical regimen. They do not seem to understand that a vigorous medical program is necessary to keep the new grafts open. Furthermore, cardiologists are concerned with the large number of people who die from coronary artery disease without even knowing they had it. Remember that 50 percent die before reaching a hospital and 25 percent die suddenly. Prevention, not surgery, is the objective.

The problems with bypass surgery are *who* and *when*. A decision for an angiogram (heart catheterization) is made after considering what risk the patient is living with and when the necessity may exist for replacing the old arteries with vein grafts to prevent catastrophe. Most often the operation is performed when the patient has such disabling chest pain that he cannot live a normal life despite all the drugs now available. The doctor must weigh the risks of performing the angiogram against the hazards of the disease. The evaluation of the exercise test, the patient's history (which is all-important), the presence of risk factors, the size of the heart, and the strength of its pumping action all figure in making this judgment.

Risk is based on the number and extent of diseased vessels. We think of the heart as having three vessels on which it depends for its vital blood supply. A vessel is considered badly diseased if its inside diameter is narrowed by 70 percent or more. If one vessel only is involved, the risk of serious heart attack or sudden death is no greater than the life expectancy of the general population, that is, around 1 to 2 percent per year. If two vessels are involved, some 6 percent will suffer a serious accident each year. If all three vessels are 70 percent or more obstructed, then the risk is at least 10 percent per year and often much higher. If the clinical evaluation and the stress test place the patient in this high-risk group, then we urge catheterization to see if he needs coronary bypass surgery (putting in veins to make new arteries) to avoid crippling heart attack or even death.

Even patients with advanced disease may do better without surgery. In my own practice, I use all the information I can get, including consultations with my colleagues, and still the decision for surgery may be difficult. After a review of their situation, some of my patients have been turned down by a conference of competent cardiologists because the disease was too extensive or the damage was already too great, or because the blood vessels did not lend themselves to bypass grafting. Still, for three years now, all of these patients except one have stayed alive—and a few are playing tennis. The one death occurred following an unavoidable prostate operation. A few of my patients who had the operation were severely crippled by their disease and died during heart surgery or shortly after; on the other hand, many with severe disabling angina have had brilliant results.

Here are two cases that illustrate how difficult it may be to know when surgery should be performed:

H. B. was a sixty-four-year-old male who was having unstable angina; that is, his pain was more and more easily provoked by exertion and particularly by emotion. At the time, he was being divorced from his wife, who was very vindictive and really didn't care whether he lived or died. His tests showed that he had three-vessel disease, and after an angiogram revealed that he had no less than 70 percent obstruction in two vessels and 85 percent blockage in his left anterior descending artery (see figure 6, page 125) he was advised to have surgery. He wasn't uncooperative, but he found it impossible to undergo such a procedure because of his divorce proceedings and because of a very lucrative business opportunity that had just presented itself. I didn't see him for eighteen months, and many times I wondered if he had died. But finally he reappeared, having spent the eighteen months in Europe. He looked fit, had lost twenty pounds, ran five miles every morning, and had lost his angina; in fact, he was taking no medicine at all. He performed a full exercise test on the treadmill with no abnormality, and stated that he had accomplished all this while experiencing great stress because of his wife, who was still suing him, and in the midst of great competition for his job!

In the next case I want to show the reader how a recognized authority on coronary artery disease goes about making these difficult decisions:

A close friend and patient of mine, W. V., had severe disease of the left anterior descending artery—the one we have referred to as carrying the highest risk—as well as major disease in another main artery. Morever, he had a large boat and often went for long trips far removed from emergency help. He had only minimal angina and had only a moderately abnormal exercise test. I sent the records to my eminent friend, Dr. Richard Gorlin, who at that time (1973) was chief of the Cardiovascular Division of Peter Bent Brigham Hospital at Harvard University Medical School. He wrote back, "I would tend to be conservative with this patient, even though I appreciate that all statistics suggest that there is an approximate 8 percent mortality in patients who have two-vessel coronary disease. All things considered, I would manage this man medically as you have done. I would without doubt encourage him to be where medical care is freely available." Bill is still voyaging on long journeys, has taken excellent care of himself, and is enjoying an enviable life without benefit of surgery.

When the arteries are severely blocked, bypass surgery can be life-saving. In general, it is necessary to consider the mortality rates in making decisions about such surgery.

It would seem that the patient with stable but severe angina and good heart function, but who has 70 percent or more of three and often two major vessels blocked is in the high-risk group and should have the benefit of surgery. A severe block in the left main and often the descending branch of the left coronary artery constitutes high risk. But attitudes are still changing as we grow in experience.

Does Surgery Improve the Quality of Life?

The term "quality of life" is often used to indicate a zest for living, the enjoyment or fulfillment of life. Survivors of bypass surgery were examined on this issue by a team headed by Dr. A. A. Rimm (Department of Preventive Medicine and Pharmacology, Medical College of Wisconsin, and Research Service Wood Veterans Administration Hospital, Milwaukee). For those men who survive heart attack and do *not* have surgery, 80 percent return to gainful employment within one year; while in the operated group, 83 percent do so. The figures are substantially the same. Other reports, some in follow-ups as long as twenty-six months, showed fewer men working after surgery than before. One study showed 82 percent unemployed. The problems of self-confidence, motivation, and physical capacity after surgery are still unsolved.

Other coronary surgical procedures have enjoyed waves of popularity. I remember when we were putting powder in the heart sac in the hope of stimulating blood flow. And doctors were just as enthusiastic about transplanting the internal mammary artery (the one that lies beneath the breastbone) directly into the heart muscle. The relief of pain was dramatic, and we were all thrilled until it was demonstrated that the same results could be obtained merely by opening and closing the chest, without transplanting the artery! It looks as though bypass is really a great operation, and in many instances, it is life-saving, but its ultimate place in the management of coronary disease will require several more years of experience and follow-up.

R. V. is a fireman who was having unrelenting chest pain of the anginal type. I was then consulting at the Sawtelle Veterans Hospital in Los Angeles. The panel of consulting cardiologists considered his case and voted for "poudrage," the operation for putting talcum powder in the heart sac. He survived the operation despite suffering another heart attack in the postoperative period. He got along fairly well for years, then had severe heart failure. Study revealed that his operation had caused scars that wrapped around his heart so tightly that it could not beat properly (constrictive pericarditis). He was saved by a lengthy and difficult operation to remove the adhesions. He is still alive and engages in a vigorous walking program thirty-years after his first operation—an operation that is no longer used.

Bypass Surgery Is Great for Severe Angina

The statistics on the results of coronary bypass surgery have recently been reviewed by Dr. J. V. Messer (Department of Physiology and Biochemistry, University of Texas Medical Branch, Galveston). First of all, he investigated what the track record for relief of heart pain was after surgery. Of patients who survived the operation, 63 percent were entirely relieved of their angina and returned to work; 16 percent were entirely relieved but were not back at work. Therefore, 79 percent had no symptoms after surgery. Nine percent had diminution of angina; 8 percent were not benefited; 4 percent were made worse or died. In general, some 60 percent had total relief, and 75 to 80 percent were improved. I think it is safe to say there is no controversy about the success of the operation in terms of relieving angina and in improving the quality of life for individuals who were suffering severe heart pain.

How many of these venous bypass grafts remain open after one year? The figure varies from 75 to 90 percent. If the circulation at the site of bypass is examined within six months, 37 percent of the vessels nourishing that area are closed off even if the graft is open; and if the graft is closed, the figure is 47 percent. If no bypass is performed, only 6 percent of this blocking will occur. This means that if the graft closes, the patient is left with no circulation in the bypassed area. These figures are improving as technical advances appear.

When a patient has all three vessels 70 percent or more blocked and is having increasing chest pain despite excellent medical management, there is no doubt that he should have surgery, often on an emergency basis. When he has a relatively undamaged heart, his mortality risk can be as low as 1½ percent in the best hands (perhaps as high as 5 percent in some less skillful ones). The relief of angina is dramatic and often complete, and the patient can return to a normal way of life, which may include sports. This is a modern surgical miracle. When the internal mammary artery is connected to the major artery on the front of the heart, the connection stays open nearly 97 percent of the time!

To keep the grafts open, however, the patient must pursue a vigorous medical and exercise regimen to combat the same factors which produced the original disease, maintains Dr. Jack Matloff, chief of cardiovascular surgery at Cedars-Sinai Hospital in Los Angeles.

With severe two-vessel disease, incapacitating angina, and a strong heart, there would still be no argument against surgery, particularly if the left anterior descending branch (on the front of the heart) was badly diseased and complete blockage would inevitably lead to sudden death or severe invalidism.

The problem of deciding whether to operate or not arises when this vessel is the only one diseased and has good flow from other vessels, or when one or two other vessels are only moderately diseased. When many such surgeries are successful, many other patients are persuaded into an operation by undiscriminating surgeons, who do not exercise the fine judgment necessary for this most important—often life-and-death—decision. And it is unfortunately true that the less the patient needed the operation, the more brilliant the result. But there are many scientific institutions such as Duke University that are searching for the truth. In their group of over three hundred matched patients, those treated medically do better than those treated surgically for the first eighteen months, and then there is little difference. But if the patients have three-vessel disease, then those treated surgically survive much longer.

These are early experiences and more data is required for firm conclusions. Other studies now indicate that surgically treated patients outlive medically treated ones. Some day the National Cooperative Study Group (National Heart and Lung Institute) and the Veterans Administration Cooperative Coronary Artery Surgery Study Groups will gather enough statistics to settle this as yet unanswered question.

How many people die from bypass surgery? The lowest mortality rate in a highly selected group is around 2 percent. The average for the country is around 4 percent.

We are living through a period of rapid advance in our abilities to diagnose accurately and to treat effectively our greatest health enemy—heart disease, particularly coronary artery disease. Our life expectancy is extended substantially every year, getting closer and closer to that nuclear time clock of at least 100 or perhaps 115 years. Surgery is great when there is no other place to turn, but even then, if you want to preserve your new arteries, you will have to do what we have been saying to prevent the need for more surgery: *Stay lean and healthy and work your heart and brain and muscles* to preserve that life force with which you were endowed.

In general, then, it may be stated that bypass surgery will not cure coronary disease or prevent further heart attack. There is insufficient evidence that it prolongs life, reduces arrhythmias, improves heart failure, improves the quality of life, or reduces the risk of sudden death. It does relieve angina and it does save lives when most or all of the arteries are severely blocked. But medical management is still preferred in the vast majority of cases—and this includes a sensible exercise program.

PART IV
For Those Who Want to Know More

By the pulsation I mean the feeling of the artery strik-
ing against the finger as it is expanded; by the pause I
mean the period of quiescence between the pulsations,
according to the length of which normal pulses are
rapid, slow, or medium. These you will determine by
the length of the pause. For a pulse is rapid when the
interval of quiescence is short, slow when the interval is
long.

Galen, 168 AD

Chapter 11.
Treadmill Exercise Test

The modern cardiologist uses the treadmill exercise test to determine a person's level of physical fitness. The treadmill, which started as a "stepping wheel," was invented in 1817 by William Cubitt and used for punishment in English prisons. By 1846, Edward Smith had adapted it to exercise testing.

With the treadmill, the physician can detect the presence of heart disease not revealed by a resting examination and can follow the response of a patient to treatment. It is recommended by the American Heart Association for anyone thirty-five years of age or older. The treadmill is now considered to be the best test used, although all tests have limitations, particularly when applied to sports medicine.

The Treadmill Test Saves Lives

The most careful history and physical examination may fail to reveal serious heart disease perhaps 50 percent of the time. It is quite true that patients have dropped dead shortly after being given a clean bill of health, but very few of these had undergone an exercise test performed by a skilled cardiologist. Even a very careful test fails to detect a certain percentage of problems, but it is very uncommon to miss a case of severe-enough disease to cause sudden, unexpected death. Every year the test is upgraded in its sensitivity and efficiency and the new tests using nuclear imaging are fantastic. Basically, it is used to evaluate the function of the heart.

How We Do It

As in other endeavors, those who perform the test frequently usually do it the best. It takes a highly trained technician or a skilled physician to carry it out properly. In our own laboratory, our chief technician, Gloria Arno, was trained in a large hospital for many years.

Then we have Peter Randaskoski, who runs our computer to assess the formidable mass of data accumulated on each test. Our apparatus includes an automatic treadmill programed to run at various speeds from 1.7 to 5 miles per hour, an automatic device for the continuous recording of blood pressure, a phonocardiograph device (for picking up the sounds the heart makes when it beats), and still another pickup which records the pulsation of an artery in the neck. These are all simultaneously recorded on a multi-channel strip writer. From these data of heart sounds, electrocardiograph, carotid pulse, and blood pressure, we have developed a profile which gives us a very satisfactory appraisal of the state of the cardiovascular system during various stages of exercise and recovery.

What We Look For

The objectives of the treadmill test may be summarized as follows:

1. To determine the level of exercise the subject can achieve, or his condition. Treadmill tests allow gradual amounts of exercise to be evaluated on the basis of the individual's tolerance. Obviously this depends on his conditioning as well as on the presence or absence of disease. Physiologists have worked out how much oxygen is burned at each level. This is like measuring the fuel consumption of your car at different speeds or revolutions per minute of the motor.

2. To determine the maximum heart rate achieved. This is most important and has many facets. As a rule, the younger the patient, the higher the heart rate that can be reached, but in sub-maximal exercise, the test is stopped when the target heart rate is reached. Conditioning and other factors determine the rate under different work loads. The "target rate" is that which should be achieved for the subject's height, weight, and age. Most tests are terminated when this level is attained. The values for the target heart rate are based on data obtained from many investigators, chiefly Dr. A. A. Bruce (authority on treadmill exercise, Department of Medicine [Cardiology], University of Washington, Seattle), but we found these often did not fit the middle-aged and older patients commonly encountered. We have revised these to fit our own population and believe they are more representative of the no-longer-young people interested in effort sports (see chapter 4, "Training Heart Rate").

If a patient has heart pain from coronary artery disease, the doctor learns at what heart rate this occurs and the patient learns his capability; and when to use his nitroglycerine and when to terminate exercise.

3. To determine the blood pressure response. Normally, the systolic (contracting) pressure should go up and the diastolic (relaxing) pressure should stay the same or drop as blood vessels dilate in the muscles. In some patients, the systolic pressure may fail to rise or the diastolic pressure rises too high. These are abnormal responses and may reveal weakness of the pumping action of the heart, high blood pressure, disease of leg arteries, or dangerous work loads for the heart patient.

4. To determine the limiting factors of exercise. What caused the patient to stop? Target heart rate reached? Excessive fatigue? Chest pressure? Irregular heart rate? Faintness? Blood pressure drop? Leg pains? Severe shortness of breath?

5. To show changes that may be indicative of disease. The electro-cardiographic response to exercise is a great diagnostic tool, but there are times when it fails to discover serious disease, or implies an abnormality that does not actually exist. The good physician must put the whole picture together to make an evaluation and is not swayed by the electrocardiogram alone (see Accuracy of Exercise Testing, page 114).

6. To determine systolic time intervals. These measurements examine the pumping abilities of the heart. The electrocardiogram is like testing the ignition system of a car, while the systolic time intervals test the power of the engine. At the same time sound recordings document abnormal heart noises. These tests are used at present only by physicians with the technical knowledge and the sophisticated equipment required. They add greatly to the total accuracy of the test, and often make a diagnosis possible in difficult cases.

7. To detect the presence of rhythm disturbances. Because they experience no symptoms when they exercise, some patients are often totally unaware that they may have a dangerous condition such as an arrhythmia. The test also helps greatly in determining whether a skip beat is harmless or dangerous (see chapter 13, "Irregular Heartbeats").

8. To follow the progress of the patient under treatment, to test the efficiency of various drugs, to test the effect of training on the cardiovascular system, to test the results of surgery, to test

recovery from a heart attack, and the like. For all these and other reasons, I consider an examination of the patient which does not include an exercise test to be most incomplete. And such a test is absolutely necessary before allowing middle-aged and older patients to play sudden-effort games like tennis.

Safety of Treadmill Test

The treadmill exercise test is remarkably safe despite its vigorous nature, and we do not hesitate to test some patients well into their sixties and occasionally in their seventies. According to Drs. P. Rochmis (of the Hygienic Disease and Stroke Program, Public Health Service, Arlington, Virginia) and H. Blackburn (professor and director of hygiene, School of Public Health, School of Medicine, University of Minnesota), the mortality rate during various types of exercise testing is 16 in 170,000 cases, or 0.009 percent. Dr. Jan J. Kellerman found that in 40,000 submaximal tests, there were no deaths within seventy-two hours. In maximal exertion in 10,000 tests, there was one patient who had a serious event after exertion, and he was successfully treated. Sometimes an irregular pulse or chest pain may be provoked by the test. If so, the test is terminated.

In office practice, the tests are always submaximal, that is, the patient is never exercised to the point of exhaustion. He stops whenever he feels he should, or if his target heart rate is reached. Obviously these tests should be conducted only by experienced people who know how to push the patient and who have the knowledge and equipment to handle untoward events.

*Not all motion is exercise to the physicians. What is
termed exercise is powerful or rapid motion or a combination of both; that is, vigorous motion with which
the respiration alters, and one begins to heave sighs. . . .*

Hippocrates, c. 420 BC

Chapter 12.
More About Exercise Testing

The electrocardiographic exercise test was given great impetus many
years ago by Dr. Arthur Masters (inventor of Two-Step Exercise Test,
emeritus clinical professor of medicine, Mount Sinai Medical Center, consultant cardiologist, Mount Sinai Hospital, New York), who used a two-
step arrangement. Later, the amount of exercise was doubled and became
known as the Double Masters Two-Step Test, but it is equivalent in terms
of work only to the 1.7-mile-per-hour level of the treadmill test, which has
replaced it in most areas. Some insurance examiners still insist on the
Masters test because they are using actuarial tables based on this test.

The Patient Usually Decides When to End the Test

The treadmill test is progressive; that is, every three minutes the speed is
increased. Starting at 1.7 miles per hour on an incline upward of a 10 percent grade, the treadmill is automatically programed to increase its speed
without pause until the test is terminated. Some patients go to 5 miles per
hour, but ordinarily a full test will terminate at 4 miles per hour (900
seconds walking time). These tests are called submaximal because the
patient's symptoms determine when the test is to stop. If the patient com-
plains of increasing chest pain, leg pain, severe shortness of breath, or exhaustion, the test is terminated. It is also terminated if the electrocardiogram shows marked irregularity, evidence of impaired blood flow, or if the
systolic (contracting) blood pressure should fall. Normally, the systolic
blood pressure elevates progressively as the diastolic (relaxing) declines or
remains unchanged. Since the pulse, blood pressure, electrocardiogram,

and heart sounds are recorded at each level, the examiner can gauge quite well how far to take the subject. Also, from much testing, there are tables to furnish a target heart rate—that rate expected for the height, weight, and age of a normal person. Most people, even though they may be unaccustomed to exercise, can reach their target heart rates.

What Is Learned

The examiner looks at the duration of exercise; the resting, peak, and ten-minute recovery heart rates; and blood pressure. He also observes the heart rhythm and notes the presence of a characteristic change in the electrocardiogram indicating diminished blood flow. This is graded according to its appearance, duration, and association with chest pain (see figure 4, page 47). In preparation for the test, the patient has gone without eating or smoking and stopped all medications which might produce false positive results; that is, cause drug-induced electrocardiographic changes that are not indicative of heart disease. An example would be a patient on a drug for the heart called digitalis or a patient whose blood potassium has been depleted by taking medicine for high blood pressure. Some unfortunate patients have been led to believe they have coronary artery disease because of such oversights. There are also patients with a peculiar conduction defect called the Wolfe-Parkinson-White syndrome, which produces false positive results in an exercise test. Or there are patients who produce a clicking heart sound which gives false test results (almost 10 percent of women).

Tests are Not the Last Word

I mention these technical matters to show that the electrocardiogram like any other test is a test and is no better than the judgment of the examining physician. In fact, if patients would understand that doctors use tests to help them find the answers to diagnostic problems but cannot rely on them as though an oracle had spoken, a lot of misunderstandings and needless anxiety could be avoided.

Figure 5. *The characteristic "ST" down-sloping displacement from the base line is the electrocardiographic change revealed by the exercise test, often with the production of angina. Under the proper testing conditions and freedom from misleading situations, this response determines the diagnosis and even the prognosis. When it occurs in many parts of the ECG and is severe, it may induce the doctor to have the heart arteries X-rayed (angiogram or coronary arteriogram) to see if bypass surgery is required.*

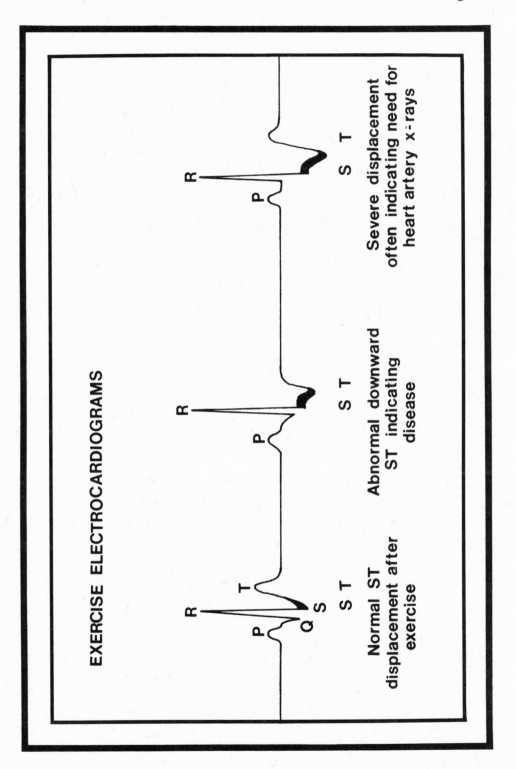

I want to point out that the electrocardiogram is a powerful tool, but even in the best hands, it can give false positive results and fail to discover disease perhaps a third of the time. It measures only the electrical pathways through the heart as they are affected by its blood supply.

Accuracy of Exercise Testing

The best way to assess the accuracy of an exercise test is to compare it with an X-ray of the heart arteries. I surveyed the reports of exercise electrocardiography in 1975 and found that up to 59 percent of the exercise tests failed to show disease. In one study of patients who had heart attacks within three to eleven weeks, 49 percent had been able to pass an exercise test! On the other hand, false positivies, that is, patients showing abnormal tests when their arteries looked normal on an angiogram, occurred in an average of 15 percent of these reports.

A new "imaging" technique is fast emerging which will greatly improve the accuracy of exercise testing and reduce the number of heart catheterizations. It is an outpatient method and consists of injecting a harmless radioactive material like technetium or thallium. These substances become "fixed" in areas of little or no blood supply, and radioactive cameras will then show them clearly.

The fact is that the exercise test *can* give false information, both positive and negative. Women in particular have many more false positive results, in which nonexistent disease is indicated. Nearly 90 percent of men with positive test results have at least 75 percent narrowing of one or more coronary arteries. Only about one-third of women with positive test results have this degree of disease in their heart arteries. If the test is negative, then the stress test is more reliable for women than it is for men; that is, there is less likelihood that the test is failing to pick up significant disease. This is because a much higher proportion of men have significant disease—53 percent versus 18 percent in women. Sometimes the patient has eaten, had a cold drink, taken drugs like digitalis, or an antihypertensive medicine that lowers potassium. Sometimes there are too few electrodes placed on the chest to show all parts of the heart.

Other Measurements Greatly Improve Accuracy

The accuracy of the exercise test can be much improved by the reading of systolic time intervals. I was one of the first to explore this field when my laboratory was supported by the National Aeronautics and Space Administration (NASA) during the Man In Space Program. At that time, NASA was searching for a way to monitor heart action other than with an electrocardiogram, because the electrical impulse can continue for some time after the heart is no longer pumping blood. We were looking not just for an electrocardiographic abnormality, but for diminished pumping action of the heart, and that is what we learn from systolic time intervals. Often they provide the clue to the presence of hidden coronary disease. Our studies and those of Dr. Richard P. Lewis have shown that systolic time intervals, added to standard treadmill exercise testing, identified coronary disease in 23 percent of patients that would have been missed by electrocardiographic evidence alone.

Electrocardiographic Error Is Greatly Reduced When Correlated with Symptoms

Although significant errors may exist, when the electrocardiographic abnormality is correlated with the patient's complaint of chest pressure, the accuracy of the test may be as high as 90 percent. In a study of 2,437 men who had no knowledge of heart disease, it was found that 85 percent of those with a positive stress test had a coronary episode in five years, while this occurred in only 2 percent of those with negative tests. I have reviewed my own patients who have gone through heart catheterization after stress testing and have found that putting together all the data that made up our profile—history; electrocardiogram; systolic time intervals; duration of exercise; and so forth—the degree of accuracy is very satisfactory.

Failure of the electrocardiogram to disclose an abnormality does not mean that the test was a poor one. The patient has to have good function to pass the test, and the diagnosis of coronary artery disease is made by a physician through evaluation of history and physical examination. All tests must be interpreted by someone with knowledge and experience.

Despite these discrepancies, as pointed out in an editorial in the *New England Journal of Medicine*, the characteristic electrocardiographic change must be regarded as evidence of disease, while realizing that it is not absolutely diagnostic, and that a negative test does not exclude disease.

Regularity and irregularity (of the pulse). . . occur in variations. By regularity is meant an even and unbroken series. For example, when the dimension of a series of pulsations continues the same, the pulse would be termed regular in size; and if the rate were unaltered, regular in rate. . .Irregularity means the destruction of even rhythm in whatever varieties of pulse it occurs."

Galen, 168 AD

Chapter 13.
Irregular Heartbeats

Arrhythmias, or irregular heartbeats, deserve special consideration in discussing the risks of exercise. Patients worry a lot about skip beats. Actually, such beats are not "skipped"—they are "premature"; that is, they occur sooner than their expected time. Some come from the small heart chambers and some from the large. Often they are not noticed, but frequently they cause palpitation, producing various disturbing but not painful sensations; a feeling of fluttering in the chest or throat, "indigestion," thumping, racing, dizziness, faintness, inability to lie on the left side, and the like. Most often they are harmless and are produced by nervous tension, coffee, tea, alcohol, tobacco, heavy meals and rapid eating which distends the stomach. Such beats are also a function of age. At age forty, about 20 percent of people have them, but at age sixty, the figure rises to 80 percent. Some people have arrhythmias all the time, even in sleep, and some only on occasion. They are classified into various categories, and are all easily identified if they are present when an electrocardiogram is being taken. We used to think they were dangerous if they appeared only during exercise, but we now know that while most tend to disappear as the heart rate increases, those that do not may still occur in healthy hearts.

Irregularities Must Be Identified

Not all irregularities are harmless. The cardiologist learns to differentiate the dangerous ones from the innocuous by noting how often they occur, if they seem to be coming from one spot in the heart or from several areas, and so on. Arrhythmias that have many of these characteristics cause sudden, rapid, irregular beating called *tachycardias*, or an irregular, rapid rhythm called *fibrillation*. When these are caused by exercise, particularly when the patient is unaware of them, they can be dangerous, even life-threatening. This is one of the major reasons exercise testing is so important. These extra beats need study, and if they are found in conjunction with known coronary-risk factors, they may indicate heart disease. But most people with skip beats do not have any disease. Again, it is necessary that a skilled cardiologist make the distinction.

The need to monitor the heart during sports activity necessitated our making portable instruments small enough to be worn without interfering with play. These gadgets have enabled us to make many observations during actual play which were not possible in the laboratory. In particular, the emotions of winning, losing, competitive instincts, and so on, are absent in the laboratory but are present during a game, and the effect of these feelings greatly influences the activity of the heart.

Detection of Irregular Heart Beats

The ability to detect abnormal rhythms during daily activities was made possible only as recently as 1961, when Dr. N. J. Holter first applied electrodes to the chest and recorded an electrocardiogram for as long as ten hours. He was able to amplify the electrical impulse from the chest wall and record it on a tape recorder. The tape was then played back through an analyzer at very rapid speeds. Thousands of heartbeats could be quickly scanned on an instrument like a television set, which would pick out the abnormal beats. It is a most useful technique, although it is cumbersome, expensive, requires many hours of operator time, is capable of misleading distortions, and sometimes fails to discover arrhythmias. Your cardiologist uses these twelve to twenty-four hour constant recordings while you keep a diary of your activities for subsequent correlations, and the data retrieved reveals the cause of many difficult-to-explain symptoms.

Patients often use words such as dizzy to mean anything from a flush to a severe disturbance of balance. Vague head sensations are variously interpreted as faintness, an awareness of a temporarily diminished blood flow to the brain, a sense of suffocation, or air hunger. Sweating, confusion, tightness in the chest, nausea, indigestion, belching, and a host of other symptoms must be studied. When these are intermittent and the office examination is negative, it is very useful to be able to correlate the changes on the Holter recording with the actual symptom when it occurs. But it may not occur during the twelve to twenty-four hour recording period of this expensive test. When no information is obtained, the test has to be repeated or other techniques used. Various remote testing systems were discussed earlier.

You may be unaware of important arrhythmias. In the past fifteen years, we have learned much from all these studies. We now know that disturbances in the rhythm of the heartbeat are very common in normal as well as abnormal hearts during average daily activities.

The decision whether to treat certain cardiac irregularities may be a very difficult one for the physician, who often has to worry about the side effects of medications, and the expense and inconvenience to the patient. In most instances, the physician can assure the patient of the harmlessness of the skip beat and allow him to live a normal life.

Arrhythmias in heart patients must be stopped. Coronary-care units have taught us that during a heart attack arrhythmias are almost universal. They are common for up to three months during the recovery period. Some deaths due to arrhythmias during this period can be avoided by control of the irregularity. Of course, the amount of physical activity allowed during the recovery period must be carefully monitored. Certainly, advanced physical exertion must not be undertaken at this time. When the patient is ready to return to normal activities, the treadmill test is often not as good as ambulatory monitoring to detect arrhythmias or to reassure an apprehensive patient about such activities as climbing stairs, having sexual intercourse, returning to work, or playing mild sports like golf. Hiking, mountain climbing, skiing at high altitudes, running, and tennis are obviously high-level activities requiring conditioning and careful study before the safety factor is established; but the fact is that many heart attack patients can participate in these activities and can even benefit from them after rehabilitation.

First of all, the auricle contracts, and in the course of its contraction throws the blood (which it contains in ample quantity as the head of the veins, the storehouse, and cistern of the blood), into the ventricle, which, being filled, the heart raises itself straightway, makes all its fibres tense, contracts the ventricles, and performs a beat, by which beat it immediately sends the blood supplied to it by the auricle into the arteries; The right ventricle sending its charge into the lungs. . .the left ventricle sending its charge into the aorta, and through this by the arteries to the body at large.

William Harvey, 1628

Appendix A
How the Circulatory System Works

The circulatory or cardiovascular system includes the heart and the blood vessels of the body; they carry blood to the tissues and then return it to the heart to be pumped around again. The blood vessels consist of arteries which carry blood away from the heart, and veins which return the blood to the heart in a closed, recirculating system. The normal human heart beats from 50 to 100 times a minute and averages about 70 times a minute at rest. That's 4,200 times an hour; over 100,000 times a day; 37,-000,000 times a year. In an average lifetime, that little muscle, no bigger than your fist, beats two to three billion times.

When the heart contracts (systole), it empties its four chambers of blood, and when it relaxes (diastole), it refills, preparatory to the next beat. At seventy beats per minute, each cycle lasts approximately 0.86 seconds or 860 milliseconds (one-thousandth of a second). Of this, the systole takes up about one-third and the diastole two-thirds of each cycle, so that the heart rests for only about a half second in each beat. Even when the heart is injured, it must go on beating. Larger animals have slower and smaller animals have much faster heartbeats.

While all this seems very elementary now, doctors did not understand the mechanism until 1639, when William Harvey (*de Motu Cordis et Sanguinis*—"On the Motions of the Heart and Blood") described his observations on circulation in animals. However, for a long time afterward, doctors continued to believe, with Galen (130−210 A.D.), the ancient anatomist,

Key to Anterior, Posterior and Cross Section Views of the Heart (pages 123, 125 and 129).

1. Anterior interventricular branch of left coronary artery
2. Circumflex branch of left coronary artery
3. Right coronary artery
4. Posterior descending coronary artery
5. Aorta
6. Pulmonary artery
7. Innominate artery
8. Left carotid artery
9. Left subclavian artery
10. Right pulmonary artery
11. Left pulmonary artery
12. Intercostal aa.
13. L. bronchial a.
14. Superior vena cava
15. Inferior vena cava
16. Coronary sinus
17. Great cardiac v.
18. Middle cardiac v.
19. Small cardiac v.
20. L. posterior ventricular v.
21. R. pulmonary vv.
22. L. pulmonary vv.
23. Opening of coronary sinus
24. Interatrial septum
25. Interventricular septum
26. L. ventricle
27. R. ventricle
28. L. atrium
29. R. atrium
30. Anterior papillary m.
31. Fossa ovale
32. Ligamentum arteriosum
33. Tricuspid valve
34. Mitral valve (bicuspid)
35. Pulmonary valve (semilunar)
36. Aortic valve (semilunar)
37. L. coronary a.
38. Anterior cusp.
39. R. coronary a.
40. L. posterior cusp.
41. L. coronary a.
42. R. posterior cusp.
43. Nodulus semilunaris
44. Sinus of Valsalva
45. Eustachian valve

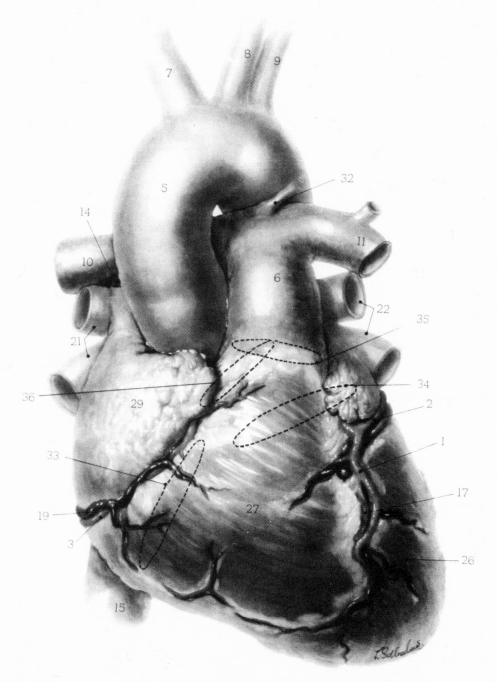

Reprinted with permission of Leon Schlossberg

Anterior

that the heart and arteries carried heat or "spirits," and did not at all realize that the heart pumps about six to seven quarts of blood around in a continuous system. The two chambers of the right side of the heart receive the blood from the great veins (the venae cavae), which return blood from the upper and lower parts of the body (see figure 6, page 127). They pump the blood through the lung arteries, which graduate from the large main (pulmonary) artery to an intricate network of tiny vessels (capillaries). These allow oxygen from the small cells of the lungs (alveoli) to diffuse through their microscopically thin walls.

The oxygen-carrying pigment of the blood—hemoglobin—picks up oxygen and unloads it in the tissues.

When the blood is laden with oxygen, the hemoglobin turns red, and when it divests itself of oxygen, it turns blue. That is why arterial blood is red and venous blood is blue. For the same reason, when a portion of the body is getting more oxygen, it is pink (the red face of blushing), and when it is returning in the small veins from tissues that have used up their oxygen, it is bluish (blue from cold).

The Blood Is an Exchange System

When the blood returns from the tissues, it has also given up its excess of carbon dioxide (CO_2), which, with water (H_2O), are the end products of tissue oxidation; that is, the utilization of energy. It is this blood that is pumped by the two left chambers through the main artery in the body (aorta) and its branches. These arteries become smaller and smaller as they get further from the heart until they are microscopic in size (capillaries), allowing only blood fluid (serum or plasma) and the tiny blood cells (white and red) to pass through. The exchange of oxygen for carbon dioxide and the exchange of foodstuff like sugar for tissue waste like urea occur at this capillary level. Here the tiny vessels are in close contact with each living cell, where all the many complex and highly specialized processes necessary for life take place. These chemical processes need not be considered here except to point out that by testing the blood for excess or deficiency of its known elements, the doctor can ascertain the presence of disease. This is why so many different blood tests are performed.

Now the blood is ready to return to the heart through the progressively larger channels of the venous system. While the arteries have muscular walls which help propel the blood, the veins are largely devoid of muscle and the blood returns passively, aided by one-way valves and the squeezing effect of the surrounding skeletal muscles.

The heart, like any other part of the body, must have a blood supply. The heart has two coronary arteries (so named because in their course

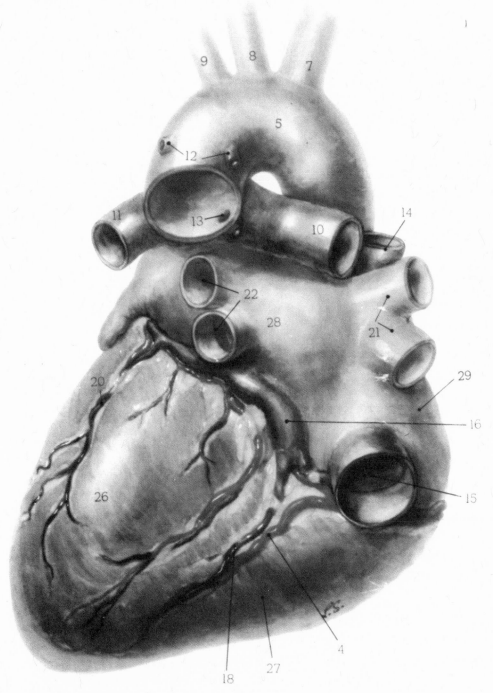

Reprinted with permission of Leon Schlossberg

Posterior

around the chambers of the heart, they resemble a crown), the right and the left. They begin at the place just after where the blood leaves the heart, through the valve of the biggest and strongest chamber of the heart (the left ventricle), and enter the aorta (this is the major arterial trunk, and like a garden hose in size and thickness). We think of the left main artery, which quickly divides as two arteries, the common trunk being only one to two centimeters long. So quickly does it branch that we think of the heart as having three major arteries.

This is important when we come to speak about disease of these arteries, because disease of one artery carries only a low risk, while disease of all three arteries is associated with a very high risk.

The left coronary artery thus divides into the major vessel, which supplies blood to the left front of the heart (left anterior descending); the other branch to the left side and back of the heart is called the circumflex. The right artery also divides into two large branches, supplying the front and back of the right heart. These vessels lie on the surface; but their smaller branches dip almost at right angles and penetrate the heart muscle, branching more and more until the first capillaries are reached—like the trunk of a tree dividing into branches and twigs until the muscle cells, like leaves, are supplied with life-giving oxygen and nourishment.

Opening and closing valves keep the blood moving forward. Since the strong muscle contraction of the heart squeezes the artery shut during systole, the blood can flow only during diastole. An additional but very small amount of blood enters the heart walls directly from the heart chambers. The blood in the heart cells is collected, as it is in other tissues, by tiny veins, poured into the large vein of the heart, and thence into the great veins of the body and recycled.

The Heart Chambers

It is necessary also to understand the functions of the small heart chambers (the atria) and their connections with the large heart chambers (the right and left ventricles). The right atrium receives blood from the two great veins which are in the upper and lower parts of the body, while the left atrium receives oxygen rich blood from the lungs. They contract nearly simultaneously, forcing blood through their respective valves into their corresponding ventricles. Therefore, when the small chambers are contracting and propelling blood through their open valves, the large chambers are relaxing and receiving blood while their valves are closed.

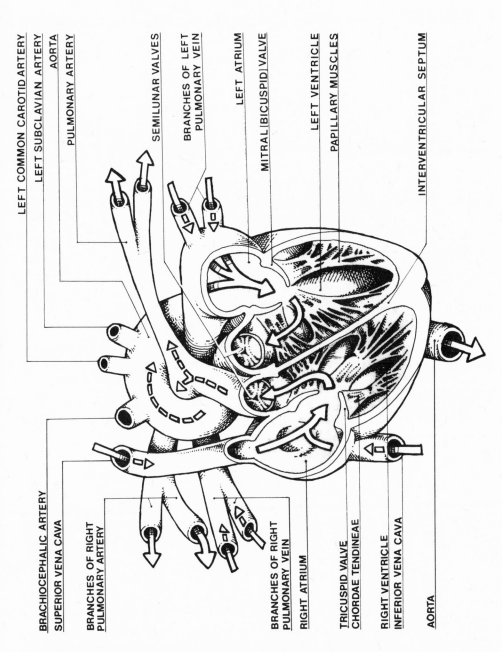

LEFT COMMON CAROTID ARTERY
LEFT SUBCLAVIAN ARTERY
AORTA
PULMONARY ARTERY
SEMILUNAR VALVES
BRANCHES OF LEFT PULMONARY VEIN
LEFT ATRIUM
MITRAL (BICUSPID) VALVE
LEFT VENTRICLE
PAPILLARY MUSCLES
INTERVENTRICULAR SEPTUM

BRACHIOCEPHALIC ARTERY
SUPERIOR VENA CAVA
BRANCHES OF RIGHT PULMONARY ARTERY
BRANCHES OF RIGHT PULMONARY VEIN
RIGHT ATRIUM
TRICUSPID VALVE
CHORDAE TENDINEAE
RIGHT VENTRICLE
INFERIOR VENA CAVA
AORTA

Figure 6. Blood Flow through the Heart

Heart Failure Can Result From Narrowed or Leaky Valves

This nicely coordinated opening and closing of gates keeps the blood moving through the chambers of the heart without any wasted energy from blood leaking back in the wrong direction. Some of the most serious heart diseases result when these valves are damaged. This can happen in two ways. The gates can become so thickened with scar tissue that they can't open easily and thus the forward motion of the bloodstream is obstructed; or the gates don't close tightly and blood leaks back in the wrong direction. In either case, and especially when those conditions are present together, the work of the heart may be so increased that even progressive enlargement of the heart eventually will result in "failure"; that is, the heart muscle gets larger in order to do more work, like any exercised muscle, but strong as it is, its limits may be exceeded and it cannot pump blood in a sufficient amount to supply the body needs.

That is what doctors mean by "failure," and it is in the prevention or treatment of valvular heart disease that the surgeon may be called upon to replace a diseased valve with an artificial one and thus extend the life of a patient indefinitely.

I have taken you on a journey as though you were a blood cell traversing the body in order to enable you to understand how the blood circulates and how the heart does its mechanical work. It is important to describe the manner in which heart motions are correlated through its ignition; that is, its electrical system (conduction system), so that you can understand the rhythm disturbances which we group under the general term of arrhythmias.

The heart has its own electrical system. In the right atrium, there is a group of specialized cells called the *sinus node*. These cells are capable of building up and discharging an electrical impulse in a rhythmic manner like a battery, the rate of which is largely determined by the action of certain substances in the blood like adrenalin, or by the influence of the nervous system.

There are brakes and accelerators in this electrical system. Two kinds of nervous fibers enter the sinus node: those from the vagus nerve are negative and slow the speed of its impulses and rate of transmission; those from the sympathetic system are positive and do just the opposite.

When the sinus node sparks, the electrical charge spreads through the atrial walls and stimulates them to contract. Next, the impulse is received by another specialized center, the atrioventricular (AV) node. From there, the charge passes through a common bundle of nerve fibers capable of transmitting electrical charges extremely fast. This bundle of nerve fibers

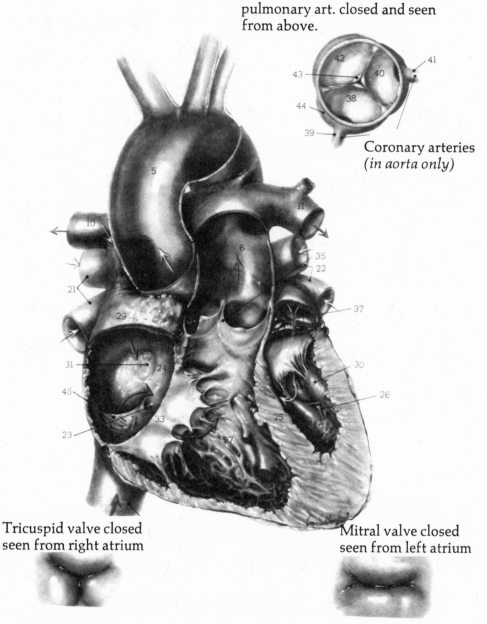

Semilunar valve of aorta and pulmonary art. closed and seen from above.

Coronary arteries *(in aorta only)*

Tricuspid valve closed seen from right atrium

Mitral valve closed seen from left atrium

Reprinted with permission of Leon Schlossberg

Cross Section

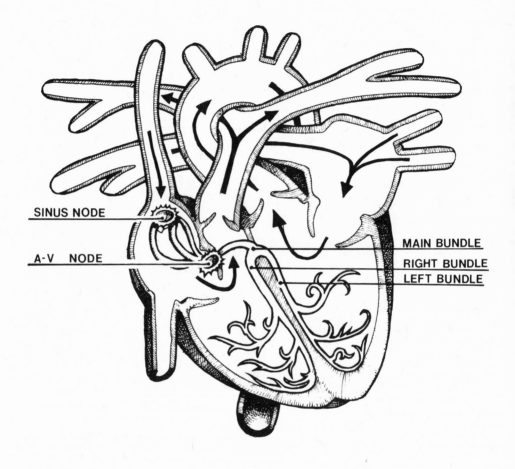

Figure 7. *The conduction system of the heart.*

Conduction nerve system of heart with origin of beat at sinus node. Main nerve bundle and right and left branches carry stimulus to all parts of heart.

Great Veins to Right Heart thru Lung Artery to Lungs.

From Lungs to Left Heart thru Great Artery to Body.

quickly divides into a right and left branch, which fan out into all portions of the large chambers of the heart and stimulate them to contract. Then the muscle rests and the process is repeated (see figure 7 on page 130).

Electrically, charges are accumulating just as though you were rubbing your shoes on a carpet, and discharging in the same way you feel a little shock when you touch something afterward. It is when the formation or transmission of this electrical system is faulty that disturbances in rhythm occur.

The Heart Is a Pump

Now that we are familiar with the blood flow, the blood supply, and the conduction system of the heart, it is time to consider its action as a pump and how it generates pressure that gives the blood its impetus to flow; that is, blood pressure.

The muscle fibers of the heart are spiraled and overlapping, so that with each contraction, the heart is "wrung out," much as you would squeeze water out of a wet towel.

With each beat, about two ounces of blood are ejected, leaving about one ounce in the major chambers. Naturally, the right and left sides must pump the same amount to maintain a balance in the lungs and the rest of the body. The pressure generated at the peak of contraction is called the systolic pressure and normally varies from around 100 to 150 ml of mercury, as measured by a blood pressure cuff over the arm artery. When the pressure falls to a few millimeters of mercury in the heart itself, it falls only to about 60 to 90 ml of mercury (diastolic pressure) in the arterial system, because the muscular walls of arteries are stretched by the systolic forces and their elasticity continues to squeeze the blood forward during diastole. Thus, the blood continues to flow while the heart is refilling preparatory to the next beat.

The Blood Pressure

Anyone can learn to measure blood pressure. One listens with a stethoscope over the bend in the elbow where the arm artery lies near the surface. The pressure is pumped by a hand bulb past the systolic pressure; then as the pressure is slowly released, a point is reached where the compressed artery begins to open and a sharp sound is heard as the blood first rushes through. This is the systolic pressure and is coordinated closely with the first bobbing movement of the mercury column, or the needle of the aneroid manometer, or feeling the pulse come through at the wrist. Then, as the pressure falls, most doctors take as the diastolic pressure the sudden disappearance of the sound made by each beat. It is very useful to learn this technique if someone in your family has high blood pressure, so as to give the doctor a much more accurate and daily account of the pressure readings.

What Happens When You Exercise

What happens to your body when you exert yourself? During activity, to provide increased blood flow to the muscles, the blood vessels increase in diameter. This may be accompanied by diminished flow to nonessential areas like the gut, and it varies with the outside temperature. Exercise in warm weather is accompanied by much more flow to the skin than in cold weather. But an area like the brain gets the same amount of blood at any level of exercise.

The heart pumps more blood by increasing its stroke output (the amount pumped with each beat), as well as by increasing its rate (the number of times it beats per minute). In prolonged heavy exercise, however, it may only be able to increase its rate. Some hearts are able to increase the amount of blood pumped per minute to seven times the amount at rest. The lungs respond by increased ventilation and gas exchange, so that the amount of oxygen consumed follows the increase in the amount of blood pumped.

Appendix B
How Things Go Wrong

Pathology means the study of disease. The purpose of this chapter is to describe in simple terms the common disease states of the cardio-vascular system so as to make clear what your physician is treating. Common diseases are those due to high blood pressure (hypertension), blockage of the heart arteries (coronary artery disease—CAD), disease of the heart valves causing obstruction of blood flow or leakage, and diseases of the heart muscle or its coverings. All of these may be associated with another group of problems, the rhythm disturbances.

Coronary Artery Disease Is the Arch Criminal

The most common heart disease is CAD. This one disease kills more people than all other causes of death put together. Every year 1,200,000 people in the United States have heart attacks and 660,000 die. Many people live long and useful lives after a heart attack, but others have heart pains—angina—and some remain permanently damaged. Figure 8 shows a normal, healthy artery and beside it a blood vessel with disease in the area through which the blood flows.

Disease narrows the channel of the artery. An artery has an outer covering wall; a middle, thick, muscular portion which can contract or dilate to change its caliber; and a very thin, perfectly smooth inner lining. A diseased vessel has a roughened lining and deposits of calcium, fat, cholesterol, scar tissue, and clotted material from the elements of the blood

Normal Artery

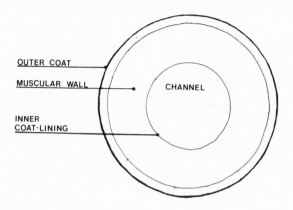

OUTER COAT

MUSCULAR WALL

CHANNEL

INNER
COAT-LINING

Diseased Artery

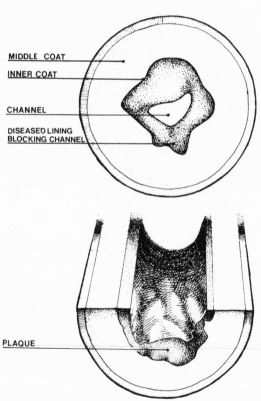

MIDDLE COAT

INNER COAT

CHANNEL

DISEASED LINING
BLOCKING CHANNEL

PLAQUE

Figure 8. *Normal artery and diseased artery showing plaque beginning to obstruct channel.*

itself, which are trapped in all this debris and are deposited on its surface as the blood flow through these portions becomes very sluggish.

A heart attack occurs when the blood flow is inadequate. Have you ever seen a bend in a winding river where the sediment is deposited as the water slows? Blood clots form in the same way when the surface of an artery is roughened, the caliber is narrowed, and the stream is greatly slowed. This disease process is very gradual and insidious, and can begin before a baby is born. Nearly all of us have some degree of these changes in our arteries as we age. In the autopsies done on Korean war veterans killed in combat at an average age of twenty-five, one-third had a significant degree of this kind of coronary artery disease. Yet many people live to old age with extensive disease because they have developed many alternate channels, which carry blood to vital areas when one or more of the vessels become plugged. In the heart arteries, if the flow is meager but still manages to support life, we call this *coronary insufficiency*. When the flow to an important vessel is shut off, we call it *occlusion*; and when so much flow is interrupted in a heart artery that the muscle supplied cannot survive, we call it *myocardial infarction* (MI). This is what people call a "heart attack," although they confuse many other sudden afflictions of the heart with this disease.

Many heart attacks go undetected. In some 18 percent of autopsies, scars of old myocardial infarctions are found—scars which were never diagnosed during life. Many of these subjects had never consulted a doctor upon experiencing discomfort. Many called it indigestion and survived without missing a day's work. I don't recommend it, but it does happen fairly often.

Everyone seems to think that a clot has to close off a heart blood vessel to cause a heart attack, but this is true probably of only a minority of attacks. In fact, the clot is more apt to follow the blockage. All that counts is whether the vessels are so diseased that the blood flow becomes inadequate to supply enough blood to the heart muscle in question. When that degree of blockage is reached—the victim may die suddenly, usually of an arrhythmia or arrest (complete stoppage). This is either asystole (no heartbeat) or ventricular fibrillation (a disorganized, weak contraction of each muscle fiber which will not pump blood). It is here that prompt resuscitation can save lives. But 25 percent of such victims die before they can receive help. On the other hand, when this occurs in a coronary-care unit, or if a trained rescue squad, like paramedics, arrive on time, the victim can be saved. The salvage rate (one-third less deaths) in a modern coronary intensive-care unit is largely due to the prompt detection and treatment of these otherwise fatal arrhythmias.

Much praise must be given to the paramedic squads who arrive so quickly. They are trained in resuscitation, carry oxygen and emergency drugs, and, of course, have immediate transportation to an emergency hospital. They can take an electrocardiogram, often read it with expertise, and possess the necessary instruments for "defibrillation": after paddle electrodes are put on the chest, an electric current jolts the quivering heart-muscle fibers into an organized, concerted contraction, which restores an effective heartbeat. But often there is no trained help around, and since time is of the essence, resuscitation must be given by the nearest available person.

The heart attack victim is usually brought to one of the coronary-care units that now exist in nearly all hospitals. Each room is equipped with special monitoring devices for recording the heartbeat, for supplying oxygen and intravenous lines for instant injection of emergency drugs. Most importantly, there are skilled nurses available around the clock who are well informed about electrocardiography, arrhythmia, emergency drugs, resuscitation, defibrillation, anticoagulation, shock, and the like. Best of all, they know how to make the heart patient comfortable and to allay his fears and those of the family. In most instances, within a few hours the patient is free of pain, relaxed, out of immediate danger, and beginning his recovery.

The development of the intensive-care unit since its initiation by Dr. Hughes Day, and the subsequent training of nurses in the skills necessary for its success, has been a truly remarkable achievement. It has been the course of medical advances throughout history that these changes came about only after overcoming the reluctance, inertia, and lack of imagination existent in many high places. I well remember having to plead with the board of my hospital when I was chief of cardiology, after a year of frustration following Dr. Day's clear demonstration in 1960 of lives saved. I remember the resistance encountered in getting our own heart association to allow nurses to perform emergency procedures and inject emergency drugs, functions previously thought to be the sole domain of the physician. And there was just as much foot-dragging about the present paramedic program, despite the impressive record which came out of Dundee, Scotland. Nevertheless, the heart associations throughout our country deserve high praise for their public educational programs and the effect these have had on reducing the mortality rate of heart attacks and strokes.

The Heart Can Never Rest

As has been shown, the injured heart must continue its work of supplying blood to all parts of the body. The objective of the physician is to reduce that work to a minimum. If you burn fewer calories by having your body perform less work, each part of the body, including the damaged part of the heart, requires less oxygen, and the work of the heart is reduced. The pulse rate then slows and the blood pressure falls.

What Happens to the Heart Muscle after Heart Attack?

It is not my purpose to describe the management of a heart attack, but I want to show that this damaged muscle needs as much rest as it can get because its blood supply is very limited, although it is not entirely absent. Some cells will die from lack of nourishment, some will survive because neighboring vessels take over the function of supplying blood. But some will die or survive depending on the delicate balance influenced by the ability to rest. This will ultimately determine the size of the scar and the amount of remaining good muscle.

At first, the muscle softens and the heart is more vulnerable to arrhythmias, even rupture in rare instances. This situation lasts for about a week, until scar tissue begins to strengthen the weakened area; by the end of the second week healing is well on its way. Many patients are sitting up in a week and go home in two to three weeks. (It was not too long ago that we kept patients flat on their backs for at least six weeks, but we know better now.)

Time Table for Recovery

By the end of the month, the patient is fully ambulatory; some go back to work in six weeks. Of course, this varies depending on the patient's age, the severity of the attack, the presence of previous or complicating disease, and the economic status of the patient. There is a saying: Two months for the poor and three months for the rich. Patients are always badgering doctors to let them do things they are not really ready to do, but often get away with. Some, however, pay the price of impatience by recurrence and extension of the damaged area, and some unfortunate ones may develop a weakened scar which is not firm enough to hold the inside pressure. Instead of contracting, this area "balloons out," or gives with each beat. This produces a very weak heartbeat and may necessitate open-heart surgery for removal of the cardiac aneurysm.

The pathology, then, is that the damaged and dying tissue is quickly replaced by scar tissue. Although a scar is left, the remaining muscle is so strong and abundant that the amount destroyed becomes unimportant in many instances and the patient can live a long and normal life. Many an afflicted person realizes that he never really knew how to enjoy life until his brush with death and his forced inactivity compelled him to contemplate the health rules he had broken and the unrewarding goals he had pursued. For the person who so changes his philosophy, the heart attack has truly been a blessing. Sir William Osler, the father of American medicine, said that the way to live a long time was to acquire a chronic disease and take good care of it.

Appendix C
Heart Rates

I examined 360 normal, healthy subjects of both sexes, ranging in age from twenty-six to seventy-eight years. They were studied while they were performing the submaximal treadmill exercise. The exercise test was terminated either by severe fatigue or by completion of five three-minute phases. Submaximal heart rates and exercise duration were evaluated to establish their relationship to age and sex. Submaximal heart rate refers only to the peak heart rate achieved and not to the subject's maximal potential heart rate. Each person was exercised to his target heart rate, the rate expected for his height, weight and age. Since age and exercise duration are also correlated, it can be seen that the maximal heart rate will vary with the duration of exercise as well, but it is primarily related to age.

To estimate the amount of oxygen burned per minute by the heart, a fairly dependable and useful rule is to multiply the heart rate by the systolic blood pressure. If you then divide by 100, you get a smaller, more understandable number. Thus, at a heart rate of 60 and a systolic blood pressure of 120: 60 x 120 divided by 100 = 72. But if the heart rate is 110 and the blood pressure is 160 systolic, then 110 x 160 divided by 100 = 176. This "double product," as we call it, can give us a fairly accurate bedside estimate of "myocardial oxygen consumption," that is, the work being done by the heart.

When a patient has anginal pain (pain due to insufficient blood flow to a portion of the heart), the double product will be about the same, regardless of the type of effort or emotion which produced it, because it represents the level at which the blood flow becomes inadequate.

Peak Heart Rates

The peak heart rate achieved during our *submaximal* test is within 10 to 15 percent of a subject's *maximum* potential heart rate.

A table of expected peak heart-rate values for each age group is given below. These are compared with maximum achievable heart rates.

Age	Target Heart Rate	Maximum Achievable Heart Rate
20	180	200
30	172	193
40	166	182
50	155	171
60	143	159
70	133	148
80	128	142

Formula for Predicted Heart Rate for Given Exercise:

$$(0.049) \text{ (Exercise Duration)} + 119$$
$$\text{(in seconds)}$$

Formula for Per Cent Maximal Heart Rate:

$$\frac{\text{Actual Maximal H R}}{\text{H R Predicted for given Exercise}} \times 100$$

or

$$\frac{\text{Actual Maximal H R}}{(0.049) \text{ (Exercise Duration)}} + 100$$

Formula for Average Training Heart Rate:

$$0.7 \text{ (Maximal H R} - 75) \quad + 75$$

Training Heart Rate: A rough estimate may be made by adding 75 at age 25 to your resting heart rate. For each five years past age 25, subtract 2 from 75. Example: You are 45. Subtract 4 x 2 (four five-year periods from age 25) from 75 = 67. Assume your resting heart rate is 64. Your training heart rate is 64 + 67 = 131 (see table page 30).

The equation for exercise duration—1,290 minus 12 x age—predicts the expected exercise duration of a normal subject given his age. A thirty-year-old patient would be expected to exercise: 1,290 − 12 x 30 = 1,290 − 360 = 930 seconds. His exercise tolerance would be considered reduced if less than 80 percent of the expected value was achieved; that is, 744 seconds. A table of expected exercise capacity and the incremental metabolic cost for different ages is given below:

Age	Expected Exercise Duration in Seconds	Exercise MPH	Calories per Minute	Metabolic Cost (METS)
30	930	4.5	14.2	12.0
40	810	4	13.0	10.8
50	690	3.5	11.0	9.5
60	570	3.5	11.0	9.5
70	450	3.0	10.7	8.3
80	330	2.3	7.8	6.5

Calorie Calculation: If you are 70 inches tall and weigh 170 pounds, you estimate that you spend 8 hours sleeping, 4 standing, 8 sitting, 3 walking, and 1 hour doing heavy work per day. The estimated basal metabolism in kilocalories* burned per hour is 71, or 1,707 per day. For sleeping you need 569; sitting, 345; standing, 1,265; walking, 773; and heavy work, 379—for a total of 3,332. If you want to lose 10 pounds in 8 weeks, you can either decrease your daily intake by 625 calories or increase your activity by the same amount. When you have reached 160 pounds you can take in 3,223 calories and maintain your loss.

Here's an example of how a scientist calculates calories:
1 liter of oxygen consumption = 5 large calories of energy
1 calorie will raise 1 kilogram of water 1 degree centigrade.
(This is one unit of heat.)
1 "large calorie" will lift 3,086 pounds a distance of 1 foot.
work = force x distance
1 foot-pound = 1 pound moved a distance of 1 foot.
1 kilogram = 2.2 pounds

METS means Metabolic Equivalents. It is the energy being burned at a basal level while awake, sitting; that is, the basal metabolic rate under these conditions. It is the equivalent of about 4 milliliters of oxygen per kilogram of body weight per minute. A 70 kilogram man will consume 70 x 4 or 280 ml/min. This is equal to 1.4 calories/min. It is the same for men of different weights. Calories are less for lighter men, more for heavier.

Aerobic Work measures the percentage of maximum oxygen consumption. This, like the percentage of maximum heart rate, varies with each in-

---

*Large or kilocalorie is the term used in metabolic studies, being the amount of heat required to raise the temperature of 1 kilogram of water 1 degree Celsius.

dividual. But they both measure the relative work of, or strain on, the heart.

Oxygen Consumption is the amount of oxygen necessary to accomplish a given work-load. It is measured in liters per minute. It will vary for persons of different weights, but if it is measured per kilogram of body weight, it will be the same for all.

Appendix D
Dr. Agress's Thirteen-Day Diet

BREAKFAST: 1st and 2nd days: 1 sliced orange, 1 cup black coffee
3rd and remaining days: ½ grapefruit, 1 cup black coffee

FIRST DAY
Luncheon: Chicken sandwich on rye toast with lettuce and tomato
Dinner: Broiled steak, celery, tomatoes, peas, sliced orange

SECOND DAY
Luncheon: Same as first day
Dinner: Broiled chicken, lettuce and tomatoes, grapefruit, tea

THIRD DAY
Luncheon: Same as first day
Dinner: Broiled steak, sliced tomatoes, grapefruit, tea

FOURTH DAY
Luncheon: 1 lamb chop, spinach, lettuce and tomato, tea
Dinner: Broiled fish, spinach and carrots, slice of fresh pineapple

FIFTH DAY
Luncheon: Swiss cheese sandwich on rye toast, ½ grapefruit, tea
Dinner Same as fourth day

SIXTH DAY
Luncheon: Minute steak, lettuce, grapefruit
Dinner Steak, peas, celery, green salad, grapefruit

SEVENTH DAY
Luncheon: Shrimp salad, ½ grapefruit
Dinner: 1 lamb chop, celery, 2 olives, carrots, peas, sliced tomato

EIGHTH DAY

Luncheon: Minute steak and tomatoes
Dinner: Steak, celery, spinach, grapefruit

NINTH DAY

Luncheon: Chicken sandwich on rye toast, juice or 1 orange
Dinner: 1 hard-boiled egg, fish, carrots, peas, celery, applesauce

TENTH DAY

Luncheon: Same as ninth day
Dinner: Broiled chicken, carrots, peas, applesauce

ELEVENTH DAY

Luncheon: Portion of sauerkraut, 2 crackers
Dinner: Steak, peas, lettuce and tomato salad, 1 slice pineapple

TWELFTH DAY

Luncheon: Swiss cheese sandwich on rye toast, tea
Dinner: Steak, peas, lettuce and tomato salad, 1 slice pineapple

THIRTEENTH DAY

Luncheon: 2 oranges
Dinner: Steak, green salad, celery, peas

All portions should be small.

All beverages should be taken without sugar or cream.

All vegetables should be eaten without butter or other dressing and little salt.

All sandwiches should be on dry toast with no butter or dressing; salads with lemon dressing if desired.

All fruits should be eaten without sugar.

Bibliography

Acker, J. E., Jr. The cardiac rehabilitation unit: Experiences with a Program of early activation. *Circulation* 44 (Oct. 1971): 119.

Agress, C. M., Arrhythmias and ischemic changes discovered during tennis not revealed by standard testing. In press.

——— Determination of stroke volume by measurement of isovolumetric contraction and ejection times. *The Physiologist* 8, no. 3 (Aug. 1965).

——— The determinants of left ventricular isovolumetric contraction time. *Japanese Heart Journal* 9, no. 2 (March 1968): 169–79.

——— Interrelationship between cardiac performance measurements. *Japanese Heart Journal* 6 (March 1966): 103–9.

——— Measurement of isometric contraction and ejection time. *American Journal of Cardiology* (March 1964): 340–48.

———Therapy of cardiogenic shock. *Progress in Cardiovascular Diseases* 6 (Nov. 1963): 236.

——— and Estrin, H. M. *The biochemical diagnosis of heart disease.* Springfield, Ill.: Charles C Thomas, 1963.

——— and Fields, L. G. New method for analyzing heart vibrations: I. Low frequency vibrations. *American Journal of Cardiology* 4 (Aug. 1959): 184–90.

——— and Fields, L. G. The analysis and interpretation of the vibrations of the heart as a diagnostic tool and physiological monitor. IRE Transactions on Bio-Medical Electronics, July 1961.

——— and Shigeo Nakakura. Measurement of cardiac events by a precise technique. *Japanese Heart Journal* 5, no. 5 (Sept. 1964): 414–430.

——— and Stroud, C. H. Heart function evaluation by real time electronic diagnosis. Proceedings of the San Diego Bio-Medical Engineering Symposium, 1961.

——— and Wegner, Stanley. Evaluation of left ventricular function in CAD by non-invasive methods. *American College of Cardiology Extended Learning Supplement* 12 (1973).

———, Wegner, Stanley, Stroud, C. H., and Bleifer, D. J. The relationship of pre-ejection contraction time to ejection time as an index of myocardial function: Vibrocardiographic correlations. *Western Society for Clinical Research* (American Federation for Clinical Research) 10 (Jan. 1962): 99.

———, Wegner, Stanley, and Schroyer, K. Thoracic transfer of cardiac energy. Proceedings of the San Diego Symposium for Biomedical Engineering 3 (1963): 24–26.

———, Wegner, Stanley, and Muller, R. M. Timing of the vibrocardiographic wave intervals for the detection of coronary artery disease. Paper read at the national meeting, American College of Cardiology, May 1961.

——— et al. Common Origin of Precordial Vibrations. *American Journal of Cardiology* (Feb. 1964): 226–31.

——— et al. Correlation of maximum O_2 consumption in athletes. *Federal Clinical Research* 10 (Jan. 1962): 99.

——— et al. The determinants of left ventricular isovolumetric contraction time. *The Physiologist* 8, no. 3 (Aug. 1965).

——— et al. Exercise test for coronary insufficiency. *American Journal of Cardiology* 9 (April 1962): 541–46.

——— et al. Indirect method for evaluation of left ventricular function in acute myocardial infarction. *Circulation* 46 (Aug. 1972): 291–97.

——— et al. Influence of heart rate on the phases of the left heart cycle in exercise. *Japanese Heart Journal* 6, no. 2 (March 1965): 104–14.

——— et al. Measurement of stroke volume. *Aerospace Medicine* 38, no. 12 (Dec. 1967).

——— et al. The normal vibrocardiogram: Physiologic variations and relation to cardiodynamic events. *American Journal of Cardiology* 8 (July 1961): 22–31.

——— et al. Signal averaging techniques for chest wall vibration recording. *Medical Research Engineering* 6, no. 7 (1967).

——— et al. Study of athletes during maximum exercise. *The Physiologist* (American Physiological Society), Aug. 1963.

Alber, Andrea J. All American sexual myths. *American Journal of Nursing* 75, No. 10 (Oct. 1, 1975): 1770.

Allen, Richard D., et al. Painless ST-segment depression in patients with angina pectoris, *Chest* 69 (April 4, 1976): 467–73.

Altschule, Mark D. Is it true what they say about cholesterol? *Executive Health* 12, no. 11 (Aug. 1976).

American College of Sports Medicine. *Guidelines for Graded Exercise and Exercise Prescription*. Philadelphia: Lea and Febiger, 1972.

Armstrong, Mark L., et al. Regression of coronary atheromatosis in rhesus monkeys. *Circulation Research* 27 (1970): 59.

Asano, T. On energy metabolism of tennis playing. *Race Hygiene* 22 (1956): 170—73.

Astrand, Per-Olof. Aerobic work capacity in men and women with special reference to age. *Acta Physiology Scandinavian* 49 Suppl. 169 (1960).

——— Effects of sports on the cardiovascular system and repercussions on the practice and health of the masses. *Schwliz. Med. Wochenschr* 104 (1974): 1538—42.

——— and Rodahl, Kaare. *Textbook of Work Physiology*. New York: McGraw-Hill, 1970, 373—430.

——— et al. Intermittent muscular work. *Acta Physiology Scandinavian* 48 (1960): 448-53.

Barnard, R. J., et al. Near maximal ECG stress testing and coronary artery disease risk factor analysis in Los Angeles fire fighters. *Cardiology Digest* (March 1976): 23—24.

Barndt, R. Jr., et al. Regression and progression of early femoral atherosclerosis in treated hyperlipoproteinemic patients. *Annals Internal Medicine* 86 (1977): 139—46.

Bar-Or, O., and Burkirk, E. R. The cardiovascular system and exercise. *Science & Medicine of Exercise & Sports*, 2d ed. New York: Harper & Row, 1973.

Barrows, Charles H. Nutrition and aging: The time has come to move from laboratory research to clinical studies. *Geriatrics* (March 1977): 39.

Bayless, Theodore M. Recognition of lactose intolerance. *Hospital Practice* (Oct. 1976): 97—102.

Benditt, D. P., and Benditt, J. M., Evidence for a monoclonal origin of human atherosclerotic plaques. *Proceedings of the National Academy of Science 70* (1973): 1753—56.

Berg, Kare, and Gorresen, A. L. Low Lipoprotein levels may raise coronary risk. *Lancet* 1 (1976): 499.

Blackburn, H., et al. Exercise tests. Comparison of the energy cost and heart rate response to commonly used single stage non-steady-state submaximal work procedures. *Medicine Sport* 4 (1970): 28.

Blocke, Antoine, et al. Sexual problems after myocardial infarction. *American Heart Journal* 90 (Oct. 1975): 536—37.

Bodansky, M., and Agress, C.M. Mortality following bilateral adrenalectomy. *Endocrinology*. 20 (Sept. 1936): 5.

Borer, Jeffrey S., et al. Electrocardiographic response to exercise in predicting coronary artery disease. *New England Medical Journal* (Aug. 21, 1975).

Boyer, John L., Director, Alvarado Medical Group Inc., San Diego, Calif. Personal Communication, May 3, 1976.

Brauer, B. M., et al. Herzgrosse und leistungs fahig keit bei tennispielern. *Theor. Prax. Korperkult* 19 (1970): 350−59.

Bruce, R.A., et al. Myocardial infarction after normal responses to maximal exercise. *Circulation* 38 (1968): 552−58.

——— et al. Seattle heart watch, initial clinical, circulatory and ECG responses to maximal exercise. *American Journal of Cardiology* 33 (Dec. 1974): 459.

Brunner, D., and Meshulam, N. Circulation in healthy old men; Medicine & Sport. *Physical Activity and Aging* 4 (1970): 80−88.

——— et al. Physical activity at work and the incidence of myocardial infarction, angina pectoris and death due to ischemic heart disease. *Journal of Chronic Diseases* 27 (1974): 217−33.

Buchwald, H., et al. The partial ileal bypass operation in the treatment of hyperlipidemias. *Advances in Experimental Medicine and Biology* 63. New York and London: Plenum Press, 1975, pp. 221−30.

Byrd, R. J., Jogging in middle-aged men: Effect on cardiovascular dynamics. *Archives of Physical Medicine and Rehabilitation* 55 (July 1974).

Carruthers, M., et al. Letters to the Editor, Safe sport. *Lancet* 1 (1975): 447.

Cassel, J., et al. Occupation and physical activity and coronary heart disease. *Archives of Internal Medicine* 128 (1971): 920−28.

Casey, Albert E., and Casey, J. G. Long-lived male population with high cholesterol intake, Slieve Laugher, Ireland. *Alabama Journal of Medical Science* 7 (1969): 21−26.

Castelli, William R. Coronary heart disease risk factors in the elderly. *Hospital Practice* (Oct. 1976): 113−21.

Chiang, Benjamin N. Relationships of premature systoles to coronary heart disease and sudden death in the Tecumseh epidemiology study. *Annals of Internal Medicine* 33 (May 20, 1974): 752−56.

Cohn, P. F., et al. Seven levels in angiographically defined coronary artery disease. *Annals of Internal Medicine* 84, no. 3 (March 1976).

Cooper, K. H. *The new aerobics.* New York: Bantam Books, 1970.

——— et al. Physical fitness levels vs. selected coronary risk factors. *Journal of the American Medical Association*, hereafter referred to as *JAMA*, 236, no. 2 (July 13, 1976): 166−69.

Craig, Timothy, T. et al. The medical aspect of sports. *American Medical Association* 16 and The Sports Medicine Foundation of America, 1977.

Davies, C. T. M., and Knibbs, A. V. The training stimulus. The effects of intensity, duration, and frequency of effort and maximum aerobic power output. Int. Z. Angew. *Physiology* 29 (1971): 299−305.

De Carlo, Thomas J., et al. A program of balanced physical fitness in the preventive care of elderly ambulatory patients. *Journal of the American Geriatrics Society* (July 1977): 331–34.

Dehn, M. S., and Mullins, Charles B. Physiologic effects and importance of exercise in coronary artery disease. *Cardiovascular Medicine* (April 1977).

Dohllof, A. G., et al. Metabolic activity of skeletal muscle in patients with peripheral arterial insufficiency. Effect of physical training. *European Journal Investigation* 4 (1974): 9.

Dolder, M. A., and Oliver, M. F. Myocardial infarction in young men, study of risk factors in nine countries. *British Heart Journal* 37/5 (1975): 493–503.

Downey, John A., and Darling, Robert C. *Physiological Basis of Rehabilitation Medicine.* Philadelphia: W. B. Saunders Co., 1971.

Doyle, J. T., Mechanisms and prevention of sudden death. *Modern Concepts of Cardiovascular Disease* 7 (July 1976).

Eckstein, R. W. Effects of exercise and coronary narrowing on coronary collateral circulation. *Circulation Research* 5 (1959): 230–35.

Edington, D. W., et al. Exercise and longevity: Evidence for a threshold age. *Journal of Gerontology* 27 (July 1972): 545.

Egeberg, O., The Effect of exercise on the blood clotting system. *Scandinavian Journal of Clinical Laboratory Investigation* 13 (1963): 8.

Ellestad, M. H., et al. Maximal treadmill stress testing for cardiovascular evaluation. *Circulation* 39 (1969): 517–22.

Engel, G. L. Sudden and Rapid Death During Psychological Stress. *Annals of Internal Medicine* 74 (1971): 771.

Erblom, B. Effect of physical training on oxygen transport system in man. *Acta Physiological Scandinavian Supplement* 378 (1969).

Faris, James V., et al. Prevalence and reproducibility of exercise: Induced ventricular arrhythmias during maximal exercise testing in normal men. *American Journal of Cardiology* 37 (March 31, 1976): 617–22.

Ferris, S. Reaction time as a diagnostic measure in senility. *Journal American Geriatrics Society* 24 (Dec. 1976): 529.

Finch, C. A., and Lenfont, C. Oxygen transport in man. *New England Journal of Medicine* 286 (1972): 407–15.

Floderus, B. Psychosocial factors in relation to coronary heart disease and associated risk factors. *Nord Hyg. Tidskr.*, Suppl. 6 (1974).

Fox, Edward L., et al. Intensity and distance of interval training with young male adults. *Medicine and Science in Sports* 5 (1975): 18–22.

Fox, S. M., and Haskel, W. L. Physical activity and health maintenance. *Journal of Rehabilitation* 32 (1966): 890.

——— Physical activity and the prevention of coronary heart disease. *Bulletin of New York Academy of Medicine* 44 (1968): 950—67.

——— et al. Frequency and duration of interval training programs and changes in aerobic power. *Journal of Applied Physiology* 38, no. 3 (March 1975).

Friedman, Meyer, and Rosenman, Ray H. *Type A Behavior and Your Heart.* New York: Alfred Knopf, 1974.

Friedman, M., et al. Instantaneous and sudden deaths. *JAMA* 225 (1973): 1319.

Froelicher, V. F., et al. Value of exercise testing for screening men for latent coronary artery disease. *Progess in Cardiovascular Diseases* 18 (Jan.-Feb. 1976): 265—76.

Goffa, D. *Los Angeles Times* (March 26, 1976).

Gottheiner, Victor. Long-range strenuous sports training for cardiac reconditioning and rehabilitation. *American Journal of Cardiology* 22 (Sept. 1968): 426—35.

Green, Andrew W. Sexual activity and the post-myocardial infarction patient. *American Heart Journal* 89, no. 2 (Feb. 1975): 246—51.

Green, Maurice R. Safety of prolonged coitus for elderly. *Medical Aspects of Human Sexuality* (July 1976): 6.

Guild, Warren R. Effect of sexual activity on athletic performance. *Medical Aspects of Human Sexuality* (July 1976): 73—74.

Guinn, Gene A., Ambulatory, nocturnal and exercise arrhythmias in coronary artery disease: A prospective randomized study to assess the influence of aorto-coronary by-pass surgery. *Cardiology* (Feb. 1977).

Gyntelberg, F. Physical fitness and coronary heart disease in Copenhagen men age 40—59. *Danish Medical Bulletin* 21 (1974): 49—56.

Hartley, H. L. Value of Clinical Exercise Testing. *New England Medical Journal* 400 (Aug. 21, 1975).

Hass, George M. Relations between human and experimental arteriosclerosis. *Modern Concepts of Cardiovascular Disease* 14, no. 3 (March 1976).

Hayflick, Leonard. The cell biology of human aging. *New England Journal of Medicine* (Dec. 2, 1976): 1302.

Hellerstein, H. K. Advances in heart disease, 1977. Paper read at San Francisco, Calif., Symposium, American College of Cardiology, Nov. 27, 1976.

——— Exercise therapy in coronary disease. *Bulletin of the New York Academy of Medicine* 44 (1968): 1028—47.

——— Techniques of exercise prescription and evaluation, in Parmley, L. F. J., ed. Proceedings of the National Workshop on Exercise in the Prevention and in the Evaluation and in the Treatment of Heart Disease, 104: *J.S.C. Medical Association* Suppl. to vol. 65 (Dec. 1969).

—— and Friedman, E. H., Sexual activity and the post-coronary patient. *Medical Aspects of Human Sexuality* 3 (March 1969): 70.

—— et al. Reconditioning of the coronary patient: A preliminary report. In Likoff, W. and Mayer, J. H., eds., *Coronary Heart Disease.* New York: Grune & Stratton, 1963, 448—54.

Herbert, Peter N. Diet and Drug Treatment of Hyperlipoproteinemias. *Audio-Digest Internal Medicine* 23 (April 7, 1976).

Herbert, Victor. The megavitamin therapy fad. *Consultant* (May 1977): 70.

Hollman, W., and Hettinger, Th. Sportmedizin-Arbeits und Trainings-Grundlagen. Stuttgart: F. K. Schattauer Verlag; New York, 1976.

Holmer, I. Physiology of swimming man. *Acta Physiology Scandinavian* Suppl. 407 (1974): 132.

I.M.C. Department of Professional Education. *One Inverness drive test.* Seminar. Englewood, Colorado.

International Society of Cardiology, Council on Rehabilitation. Myocardial infarction: How to prevent, how to rehabilitate. 1973.

Ippoliti, Andrew F. The effect of various forms of milk on gastric acid secretion. *Annals of Internal Medicine* 84 (March 1976): 286—89.

Jenkins, David C. Psychologic and social risk factors for coronary disease. *New England Journal of Medicine* 29 (April 29, 1976): 982—94.

Jobaris, Russel, et al. Duration of orgasm. *Medical Aspects of Human Sexuality* (July 1976): 7.

Johnson, L. C., and O'Shea, J. P., Anabolic steroids: Effect on strength development. *Science* 164 (May 23, 1969): 567.

Jokl, Ernst, et al. Advances in exercise physiology. *Medicine and Sports* 9 (1976).

—— *Physical Activity and Aging.* Baltimore, Md.: University Park Press, 1970.

—— The contribution of sports medicine to clinical cardiology. *American Correspondent Therapeutic Journal* (May—June 1975).

—— and McClellan, J. T. Exercise and cardiac death. *Medicine and Sport* (1971).

Jukes, Thomas H. Food Additives. *New England Journal of Medicine* 297 no. 8 (Aug. 27, 1977): 427—430.

Kannel, William B. Some lessons in cardiovascular epidemiology from Framingham. *American Journal of Cardiology* 37 (Feb. 1976): 269—82.

—— Habitual level of physical activity and risk of coronary heart disease. Proceedings of the International Symposium on Physical Activity and Cardiovascular Health. *Canadian Medical Association Journal* 96 (1967): 811.

—— and Sorlie, Paul. Remission rates for angina pectoris: 20-year follow-up. The

Framingham study. *American Journal of Cardiology* (Feb. 1977): 2870.

——— et al. A General Cardiovascular risk profile: The Framingham Study. *American Journal of Cardiology* 38 (July 1976): 46—51.

——— et al. Precursors of sudden coronary death: Factors related to the incidence of sudden death. *Circulation* 51/4 (1975): 606—13.

Kasch, Fred W. Rope skipping offers a good aerobic alternative. *The Physician and Sports Medicine* 122 (April 1976).

Kasser, I. S., and Bruce, A. A. Comparative effects of aging and coronary artery disease on submaximal and maximal exercise. *Circulation* 44 (1971): 759—74.

Kattus, A. A., et al. ST-segment depression with near maximal exercise in detection of preclinical coronary heart disease. *Circulation* 44 (1971): 585—95.

Kavanaugh, Terrence. Interval training of the post-coronary patient. *Archives of Physical Medicine and Rehabilitation.* 56 (Feb. 1975): 72.

——— and Shepard, Ray H. Maximal exercise tests on post-coronary patients. *JAMA* 229 (April 29, 1976): 982—94.

Karvonen, M. J., et al. Longevity of endurance skiers. *Medicine & Science in Sports* 6 (1974): 49—56.

Kellerman, Jan J. Rehabilitation of patients with coronary heart disease. *Progress in Cardiovascular Diseases* 17 (Jan.—Feb. 1975).

Kent, Saul. What's behind the dramatic increase in cardiovascular mortality with aging? *Geriatrics* 31 (Sept. 1976): 134.

Keys, A. Physical activity and the epidemiology of coronary heart disease, in D. Brunner and E. Jokl, eds., *Internal Medicine and Sport* 4 (Baltimore, Md., University Park Press, 1970): 250—66.

Kilbourn, A., et al., Physical training in sedentary middle aged and older men. *I. Medical Evaluations Scandinavian Journal Clinical Laboratory Investigations* 24 (1969): 315—34.

Knibbs, A. V., et al. Anabolic effects of methandrostenolone in men undergoing athletic training. *Lancet* 11 (Oct. 2, 1976): 699.

Knipping, H. W. Uber die Funktionsprieting Von Herz and Kreislauf. *Beitrogen Klinische* 88 (1937): 95.

Knuttgen, H.G. Physical conditioning through interval training with young male adults. *Medicine and Science in Sports* 5 (1973): 220—26.

Kraus, H. and Raab, W. *Hypokinetic disease: Diseases produced by lack of exercise.* Springfield, Ill.: Charles C Thomas, 1961.

Kuller, N. Coronary artery disease: Cause of three-out-of-four deaths in unconditioned joggers. *American Journal of Cardiology* 24 (1969): 617.

Leaf, Alexander. *Youth in old age.* New York: McGraw-Hill, 1974.

Lehman, H. C. *Science* 98 (1943): 270—73.

Lewis, Richard P. et al. Usefulness of systolic time intervals in coronary artery disease. *American Journal of Cardiology* 37 (April 1976): 787–96.

Librach, Gershon, et al. Stroke: Incidence and risk factors. *Geriatrics* (April 1977).

Licht, Sidney, and Johnson, Ernest W. *Therapeutic exercise*. Baltimore: Waverly Press, 1965.

Lim, J. S., Proudfit, W. L., and Sones, F. M., Jr. Left main arterial obstruction: Long term follow-up of 141 nonsurgical patients. *American Journal of Cardiology* 36 (1975): 131–35.

Lintgen, Arthur B. Death from myocardial infarction after exercise test with normal result. *JAMA* 235, no. 8 (Feb. 23, 1976): 837–39.

Lown, Bernard, and Verrier, Richard L. Neural activity and ventricular fibrillation. *New England Journal of Medicine* 294, no. 21 (May 20, 1976).

——— and Graboys, Thomas B. Sudden Death: An Ancient Problem Newly Perceived. *Cardiovascular Medicine* 2, no. 3 (March 1977): 219.

Luke, J. L., and Halpern, M. Sudden and unexpected death from natural causes in young adults: Review of 275 consecutive autopsied cases. *Archives Pathology* 85 (1968): 10–17.

Mann, George V. Diet and obesity. *New England Medical Journal* (April 7, 1977): 812.

Mann, G. U., Garrett, L., and Long, A. The amount of exercise necessary to achieve and maintain physical fitness in adult persons. *Southern Medical Journal* 64 (1971): 549–53.

Master, A. M., and Jaffe, H. L. Factors in the onset of coronary occlusion and coronary insufficiency: Effort, occupation, trauma and emotion. *JAMA* 148 (1952): 794.

Masters, W. H., and Johnson, V. E. *Human sexual response*. Boston: Little, Brown, 1966.

McAlpin, R. B., and Kattus, A. A. Adaptation to exercise in angina pectoris. *Circulation* 33 (1966): 183.

McHenry, Malcolm M. Medical screening of patients with coronary artery disease. *American Journal of Cardiology* 33 (May 20, 1974): 752–56.

Mead, Wm. F. Exercise rehabilitation after myocardial infarction. *AFP* (March 1977): 121–26.

Medalie, Jack H., and Goldbourt, U. Unrecognized myocardial infarction. 5-Year incidence, mortality and risk factors. *Annals of Internal Medicine* 84 (1976): 526–31.

——— et al. Angina pectoris among 10,000 men. *American Journal of Medicine* 55 (1973): 583–94.

Medical World News (Nov. 1, 1976): 52–57. Giving up smoking: How the various programs work.

Merriman, J. E. The physiologic effects of physical activity in cardiac patients. *Acta Cardiological Supplement* 14 (1970): 39–46.

Messer, J. V. Coronary artery bypass surgery. *Audio Digest, Internal Medicine* 23, no. 3 (Feb. 2, 1976).

Mitchell, J. H. Exercise training in the treatment of coronary heart disease. *Advances in Internal Medicine* 20 (1975): 249.

——— et al. Vigorous exercise in leisure time and the incidence of coronary heart disease. *Lancet* 1 (1973): 333.

Morris, J. N., and Crawford, M. D. Coronary heart disease and physical activity of work evidence of a natural necropsy survey. *British Medical Journal* 2 (1950): 1485–96.

Morse, Robert L. *Exercise and the heart.* Springfield, Ill.: Charles C Thomas, 1972.

Mortimer, Edward A. Jr., et al. Reduction in mortality from coronary heart diease in men residing at high altitude. *New England Journal of Medicine* (March 17, 1977).

Mulcahy, Risteard. Factors influencing long-term prognosis in patients with coronary disease. *Cardiology Digest* (Nov. 1976): 11.

The multiple risk factor intervention trial. *JAMA* 235, no. 8 (Feb. 23, 1976): 825.

Murphy, Marvin L., et al. Surgical versus medical therapy for coronary artery disease, survival data: Preliminary report of the VA cooperative study. *American Journal of Cardiology* (Feb. 1977): 286.

Naughton, John P., and Hellerstein, Herman K. *Exercise testing and exercise training in coronary heart disease.* New York: Academic Press, 1973.

Nemec, E. D., et al. Heart rate and blood pressure responses during sexual activity in normal males. *American Heart Journal* 92 (Sept. 1976): 274–77.

Nichols, Allen B., et al. Independence of serum lipid levels and dietary habits. The Tecumseh Study. *JAMA* 246, no. 17 (Oct. 25, 1976).

Norman, John C. *Coronary artery medicine & surgery: Concepts & controversies.* New York: Appleton-Century Crofts.

Ochsner, Alton. Aging. *Journal of American Geriatrics Society* 24, no. 9 (Sept. 1976).

Opie, Lionel H. Exercise training, the myocardium and ischemic heart disease. *American Heart Journal* 88, no. 5 (Nov. 1974).

——— Sudden death and sport. *Lancet* 1 (Feb. 1, 1975): 263–66.

Paffenbarger, R. S., Jr., and Hale, W. E. Work activity and coronary heart mortality. *New England Journal of Medicine* 292 (1975): 545.

Passmore, R., and Durmin, J. V. Human energy expenditure. *Physiological Review* 35 (1955): 801.

Pauget, J. M., et al. Abnormal responses of systolic time intervals to exercise in patients with angina pectoris. *Circulation* 43 (1971): 289.

Petro, J. K., et al. Instantaneous cardiac acceleration in man induced by a voluntary muscle contraction. *Journal of American Physiology* 29 (1970): 794.

Pettyjohn, F. S., and McKeekin, R. R. Coronary artery disease and preventive cardiology in aviation medicine. *Aviation, Space and Environmental Medicine* 46 (1975): 1299–1304.

Pfeiffer, Eric. Sexuality in the aging individual. *American Geriatrics Society* 22 (11) (Nov. 1974): 481–84.

Pribble, A. Failing exercise testing to detect ventricular artery hernias. *Clinical Research* 23 (1975): 125A.

——— et al. Failure of exercise testing to detect ventricular arrhythmias. *Clinical Research* 23 (1975): 125A.

Pollock, M. L. et al. Physiologic responses of men 49 to 65 years of age to endurance training. *American Geriatrics* Society 24, no. 3 (March 1976).

——— et al. Effects of training two days per week at different intensities on middle aged men. *Medical Science Sports* 4 (1972): 192.

Pyfer, H. R., and Doane, B. L. Cardiac arrest during exercise testing. *JAMA* 210 (1969): 101–02.

——— et al. Exercise Rehabilitation in Coronary Heart Disease: Community Group Programs. *Archives of Physical Medicine and Rehabilitation* 57 (July 1976).

Quint, Jules V., and Cody, B. R. Preeminance and mortality: Longevity of prominent men. *British Medical Journal* 60 (Aug. 24, 1974): 118–24.

Rabkin, Simon W. Relation of body weight to development of ischemic heart disease in a cohort of young North American men after a 26 year observation period: The Manitoba study. *American Journal of Cardiology* 39 (March 1977): 452.

Raskoff, Wm. J., et al. The athletic heart prevalence and physiological significance of left ventricular enlargement in distance runners. *JAMA* 236, no. 2 (July 12, 1976): 158–161.

Rechnitzer, P. A., et al. Long term follow-up study of survival and recurrence rates following myocardial infarction in exercising and control subjects. *Circulation* 45 (1972): 853–57.

Redwood, D. R., et al. Circulatory and symptomatic effects of physical training in patients with coronary artery disease and angina pectoris. *New England Journal of Medicine* 286 (1972): 959–65.

Rhoads, George G. et al. Serum lipoproteins and coronary heart disease in a population study of Hawaiian and Japanese men. *New England Journal of Medicine* 294 (1976): 293.

Rimm, A. A., et al. Changes in occupation after aortocoronary vein bypass operation. *JAMA* 236, no. 4 (July 26, 1976): 361.

Rochmis, P., and Blackburn, H. Exercise tests: A survey of procedures, safety and litigation experience in approximately 170,000 tests. *JAMA* 217 (1971): 552–58.

Rose, G., et al. Myocardial infarction and the intrinsic calibre of coronary arteries. *British Heart Journal* 29 (1967): 548–52.

Rosenman, R. H., Friedman, M., et al. Coronary heart disease in the Western collaborative group studies in follow-up experience of two years. *JAMA* 195 (1966): 80–92.

——— et al. Multivariate prediction of coronary heart disease during 8.5 year follow-up in the Western collaborative group. *American Journal of Cardiology* 37 (May 1976): 903–10.

Roshamen, H. Optimum pattern of exercise for healthy adults. *Canadian Medical Association Journal* 96 (1967): 895.

Rusk, Howard A. *Rehabilitation Medicine.* New York: C. V. Mosby Co., 1971.

Saltin, B., et al. Physical training in sedentary middle-aged and older men. *Scandinavian Journal of Clinical Laboratory Investigation* 24 (1969): 323–34.

Scaff, Jack H., Heart disease in marathon runners. *New England Journal of Medicine* 295, no. 2 (July 8, 1976): 105.

Schaper, W., et al. Der einfluss korperlichen trainings auf den bilateral kreislauf des herzen verk. *Germany Kreise-Forsch* 37 (1971): 112.

Scheuer, J. Physical training and intrinsic cardiac adaptations. *Circulation* 42 (1973): 677.

Schiffer, Frederic, et al. The quiz electrocardiogram. *American Journal of Cardiology* 37 (1976): 41–47.

Seliger, V., et al. Energy metabolism in tennis. Intimal Zeitscheift Angewissenschaft. *Physiology* 31 (1973): 333–40.

Sharmas, et al. Raw or cooked onions may improve serum cholesterol. *Indian Journal of Nutritious Diet* 12 (1975): 288.

Shephard, R. J., Current view of Canadian fitness. *Canadian Family Physician* 19 (1973): 57.

Shock, N. W., and Norris, A. H. Neuromuscular coordination as a factor in age changes in muscular exercise. *IBID* (1970): 92–99.

Sketch, Michael H., and Turner, David A. Sex differences in stress testing. *American Journal of Cardiology* 38 (July 1976): 135–38.

Spodick, D. H. Aortocoronary bypass surgery for ischemic heart disease: Indications based on control trials. *Postgrad Medicine* 59: 70–3.

Stark, R. S., et al. Left ventricular performance in coronary artery disease evaluated with systolic time intervals and echocardiography. *American Journal of Cardiology* 37 (March 4, 1976): 331.

Stein, Richard A. Effect of exercise training on heart rate during coitus in the post-myocardial infarction patient. *Circulation* 51 and 52 (Oct. 1975).

Taylor, H. T., et al. Death rates among physically active and sedentary employees of the railroad industry. *American Journal of Public Health* 52 (1962): 1697–1707.

Thomas, C. B. Precursors of Premature Disease and Death. *Annals of Internal Medicine* 85 (1976): 653–58.

Vaisrub, Samuel, Quality of life manqué. *JAMA* 236, no. 4 (July 26, 1976): 387.

Varnouskas, E. M. et al. Peripheral hemodynamic effects of physical health and in ischemic heart disease. *Ischemic Heart Disease Leyder* 219 (1970).

Vasta, et al. Regression of stenotic lesions of renal arteries and spontaneous cure of hypertension. *American Journal of Medicine* vol. 7, 1977.

Vismara, L. A., and Mason, D. T. Relation of ventricular arrhythmias in late hospital phase of acute myocardial infarction to sudden death after hospital discharge. *American Journal of Medicine* 59 (1975): 6–12.

Vitamin E: Miracle or myth? *Nutrition Review* Suppl. 35, 32 (July 1974): 35 (reprint of FDA *Consumer*, Department of Health, Education and Welfare, July-August 1973).

Vitamin E supplement and fatigue. *New England Journal of Medicine* 290 (March 7, 1974): 579 (letter to the editor).

Walker, Weldon J. Curbing risk factors has helped reduce U.S. coronary deaths. *Modern Medicine* 44 (June 1, 1976): 33–47.

Wenger, N. C. The use of exercise in the rehabilitation of patients after myocardial infarction. *J.S.C. Medical Association* 65, Supp. 1 (1969): 66–8.

Whitsett, T. L., and Naughton, J. P. The effect of exercise on systolic time intervals in sedentary and active individuals and rehabilitated patients with heart disease. *American Journal of Cardiology* 27 (1971): 352.

Whyte, H. M. Potential effect on coronary heart disease morbidity of lowering blood cholesterol. *Lancet* 1/7912 (1975): 447.

Wilmore, Jack H. Individual exercise prescription. *American Journal of Cardiology* 33 (May 20, 1974): 757–60.

Wissler, Robert W., and Vesselinovitch, Dragoslava. Regression of atherosclerosis in experimental animals and man. *Modern Concepts of Cardiovascular Disease* 46 (June 1977): 27–32.

Wright, Irving S. Correct levels of serum cholesterol. *JAMA* 236, no. 2 (July 12, 1976): 261–62.

Wyatt, H. L., and Mitchell, J. H. Influences of physical conditioning and deconditioning upon the coronary vasculature of dogs. *American Journal of Cardiology* 39 (Feb. 1977): 262.

Wyndham, C. H., and Ward, J. S. An assessment of the exercise capacity of cardiac patients. *Circulation* 16 (1957): 384.

Xenakis, Alan P., et al. Instantaneous cardiac acceleration in man induced by a voluntary muscle contraction. *Journal of American Physiology* 29 (1970): 794.

Yano, Katsuiko, et al. Coffee, alcohol and risk of coronary heart disease among Japanese men living in Hawaii. *New England Journal of Medicine* 297 (Aug. 25, 1977): 406–09.

Young, R. L., et al. Chorionic gonadotropin in weight control, a double-blind crossover study. *JAMA* 236, no. 22 (Nov. 29, 1976): 2495–97.

Zukil, W. J., et al. A short-term community study of the epidemiology of coronary heart disease: A preliminary report on the North Dakota study. *American Journal of Public Health* 49 (1959): 1630–39.

Index